The Significance of Touch in Psychiatry

The Significance of Touch in Psychiatry

Clinical and Neuroscientific Approaches

Editors

Bruno Müller-Oerlinghausen
Michael Eggart

MDPI • Basel • Beijing • Wuhan • Barcelona • Belgrade • Manchester • Tokyo • Cluj • Tianjin

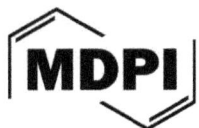

Editors
Bruno Müller-Oerlinghausen
Charité Universitätsmedizin
Berlin
Germany

Michael Eggart
Hochschule Ravensburg-
Weingarten University of
Applied Sciences
Germany

Editorial Office
MDPI
St. Alban-Anlage 66
4052 Basel, Switzerland

This is a reprint of articles from the Special Issue published online in the open access journal *Actuators* (ISSN 2076-0825) (available at: https://www.mdpi.com/journal/brainsci/special_issues/ Touch_Neuroscientific).

For citation purposes, cite each article independently as indicated on the article page online and as indicated below:

LastName, A.A.; LastName, B.B.; LastName, C.C. Article Title. *Journal Name* **Year**, *Volume Number*, Page Range.

ISBN 978-3-0365-0382-0 (Hbk)
ISBN 978-3-0365-0383-7 (PDF)

© 2021 by the authors. Articles in this book are Open Access and distributed under the Creative Commons Attribution (CC BY) license, which allows users to download, copy and build upon published articles, as long as the author and publisher are properly credited, which ensures maximum dissemination and a wider impact of our publications.

The book as a whole is distributed by MDPI under the terms and conditions of the Creative Commons license CC BY-NC-ND.

Contents

About the Editors . . . . **vii**

Bruno Müller-Oerlinghausen and Michael Eggart
Touch Research–Quo Vadis? A Plea for High-Quality Clinical Trials
Reprinted from: *Brain Sci.* **2021**, *11*, 25, doi:10.3390/brainsci11010025 . . . . **1**

Michaela Maria Arnold, Bruno Müller-Oerlinghausen, Norbert Hemrich and Dominikus Bönsch
Effects of Psychoactive Massage in Outpatients with Depressive Disorders: A Randomized Controlled Mixed-Methods Study
Reprinted from: *Brain Sci.* **2020**, *10*, 676, doi:10.3390/brainsci10100676 . . . . **7**

Rebecca Boehme, Helene van Ettinger-Veenstra, Håkan Olausson, Björn Gerdle and Saad S. Nagi
Anhedonia to Gentle Touch in Fibromyalgia: Normal Sensory Processing but Abnormal Evaluation
Reprinted from: *Brain Sci.* **2020**, *10*, 306, doi:10.3390/brainsci10050306 . . . . **25**

Sabine B.-E. Baumgart, Anja Baumbach-Kraft and Juergen Lorenz
Effect of Psycho-Regulatory Massage Therapy on Pain and Depression in Women with Chronic and/or Somatoform Back Pain: A Randomized Controlled Trial
Reprinted from: *Brain Sci.* **2020**, *10*, 721, doi:10.3390/brainsci10100721 . . . . **39**

Anita Ribeiro Blanchard and William Edgar Comfort
Keeping in Touch with Mental Health: The Orienting Reflex and Behavioral Outcomes from Calatonia
Reprinted from: *Brain Sci.* **2020**, *10*, 182, doi:10.3390/brainsci10030182 . . . . **53**

Bernhard Reichert
Does the Therapist's Sex Affect the Psychological Effects of Sports Massage?— A Quasi-Experimental Study
Reprinted from: *Brain Sci.* **2020**, *10*, 376, doi:10.3390/brainsci10060376 . . . . **71**

About the Editors

Bruno Müller-Oerlinghausen, Prof.em. of Clinical Psychopharmacology, at Charité-Universitätsmedizin, Berlin (Germany) is a specialist Clinical Pharmacology. He was born in Berlin; after taking the state examination for medicine he began a postgraduate training in pharmacology and toxicology at the University of Göttingen (1964–1969). From 1969 to 71, he was assigned a foreign aid project at the Dept. of Medical Science (Ministry of Public Health) in Bangkok, Thailand. In 1971, he began additional training in clinical psychiatry at the Freie Universität of Berlin. In 1974, he was promoted to Prof. of Clinical Psychopharmacology and as the Chief Scientist of a specialized outpatient clinic for the long-term care of patients with affective disorders (Berlin Lithium Clinic). From 1983 to 87, he acted as President of the German Association of Neuropsychopharmacology (AGNP). From 1994 to 2007, he was the acting chairman of the Drug Commission of the German Medical Association. His international research was primarily devoted to the long-term effects of lithium under special consideration of its antiaggressive, antisuicidal and serotonergic effects. Since 1998 he has taken a strong interest in the effects of complementary therapies, especially body-focused treatments. He conducted the first controlled study on the antidepressive effects of Slow Stroke massage, followed by further research projects and publications on touch therapies. In 2004, he received a research award by the American Foundation for Suicide Prevention. In 2007, he was honoured with the Paracelsus Medal, the highest-ranking award of the German Medical Association, conferred by Deutsche Ärztetag.

Michael Eggart studied Applied Health Sciences at the Ravensburg-Weingarten University of Applied Sciences and graduated with a master's degree in 2017. He is currently a doctoral student at the Medical Faculty of Ulm University, Department of Psychiatry and Psychotherapy I, Germany. His research interests include the relationship between interoception and mental health, psychophysical effects of interpersonal touch and the underlying mechanisms of touch therapies in affective disorders.

Editorial

Touch Research–Quo Vadis? A Plea for High-Quality Clinical Trials

Bruno Müller-Oerlinghausen [1],* and Michael Eggart [2]

1. Charité Universitätsmedizin Berlin, 10117 Berlin, Germany
2. Faculty Social Work, Health and Nursing, Ravensburg-Weingarten University of Applied Sciences, 88250 Weingarten, Germany; michael.eggart@rwu.de
* Correspondence: bruno.mueller-oerlinghausen@web.de

Recently, the issue of a lack of interpersonal touch has gained much public interest due to the social distancing ordered by the authorities in the present pandemic situation [1]. Discussions on the social and medical value of touch nowadays will not be restricted to the realm of sociology, psychotherapy or philosophy but can refer to the ongoing and steadily increasing international research on the effects of touch in animals and humans and their underlying biological mechanisms [2]. It is largely to the credit of Swedish researchers that a new and fascinating branch of research has emerged within the last two decades, e.g., through the exploration of particular unmyelinated nerve fibers in the non-glabrous skin that specifically respond to gentle, interpersonal touch mediating feelings of well-being. From an epistemological point of view, it is noteworthy that the discovery of the so-called C tactile afferents (CT) in mammalians coincided with the emergence of social neuroscience in the early 1990s, probably marking a paradigm shift in the life sciences. In this respect, neurophysiologists have coined the term "affective touch", which relates to both affection through skin-to-skin contact and positive affective states that are elicited by the touch experience [2]. Considering interpersonal touch from the bottom-up, the affiliative nature of affective touch is mainly, but probably not exclusively mediated by the CT system in the non-glabrous skin projecting to brain regions, which have been associated with social reward and interoception. However, a comprehensive understanding of social touch also includes top-down processes involving contextual factors that shape the touch experience, mainly represented by (a) the person giving touch ("who") and (b) the underlying intention ("why") [3]. Interestingly, the term "affective touch" was already used in the context of research into nursing in the 1980s and referred to touch experiences that are not task-related but can satisfy the basic human need for touch [4].

Many studies have explored the effects of various kinds of affective touch on the nervous system as well as on various neuropeptides such as oxytocin, stress hormones, the vagal tone, immunological parameters, etc. [5]. Recent studies have also investigated the neural processing of affective touch in mental disorders (see, e.g., [6] in this Special Issue). However, the introduction of specified touch techniques, e.g., psychoactive massage therapy into the treatment of psychiatric illness such as depression, anxiety or psychosomatic disorders as well as chronic pain, e.g., in patients with cancer [7], still meets much skepticism or open resistance often revealing stupendous ignorance of the existing scientific findings.

In the following, we are going to present some arguments why therapeutic touch should find its place within the multimodal therapy of particularly affective disorders. We shall particularly present our personal views on what kind of clinical studies in this area should be designed and performed in the future. This discussion will also touch on certain elements of the original articles collected in this Special Issue of *Brain Sciences*, which we had the pleasure and honor to edit.

Why do we need more and novel therapeutic approaches to the area of affective disorders? So far, the main treatments of depressed patients consist of either antidepressant drugs or psychotherapy. However, their general effectiveness is limited and far from satisfactory. This refers not only to the use of antidepressants, whose steadily increasing use and the spectrum of adverse drug reactions have provoked critical voices, but also to cognitive behavioral psychotherapy and mindfulness techniques. Their overall efficacy might also have been overestimated in the past [8–12]. Accordingly, it has been shown that one third of patients still present with residual symptoms at the end of treatment, which have been linked to worse long-term outcomes by predicting recurrent depression and significantly reducing quality of life [13]. Thus, an urgent need exists for the development of new and safe treatments for this indication, which are also accepted by the inflicted patients. It might be an interesting signal that particularly depressed patients and among them often women seek help from complementary treatments, and among them especially all kinds of massage [14]. In fact, some earlier and more recent systematic literature surveys including a meta-analysis of existing clinical studies strongly support the effectiveness of various kinds of massage in depressed patients in spite of various methodical deficits and particularly the heterogeneity of the studies performed so far [15–17].

What can be done in the future on behalf of academic medicine, clinical psychology, and basic research to make touch therapies attractive and an accepted treatment option for psychiatric or psychosomatic patients? We argue that a broader acceptance of touch in medicine will only be achieved on the basis of valid and high-quality scientific studies. There are, however, some important requirements, which should be met in future studies and scientific approaches.

First of all, we are in need of excellent clinical studies comparing the mental and somatic effects and particularly anti-depressive efficacy of various kinds of affective touch, e.g., realized as psychoactive massage vs. established body-focused treatments such as relaxation methods, aerobic/anaerobic training, mind-body techniques, etc. It should be clarified whether and if so in which respect will the effects of massage using affective, gentle touch differ from those of classical (Swedish) massage in patients with affective or psychosomatic disorders. The applied manual techniques have to be described precisely (see, e.g., [18,19]), a postulate that has already been brought forward in various reviews [15,16]. Accurate description of the applied methods is also important, since some authors have argued that moderate pressure and not exclusively light stroking is required to obtain useful therapeutic effects. This argument has been brought forward particularly against the background of the hypothesis that it is the increased vagal tone, which explains the observed therapeutic effects, also, e.g., on the immune system [5]. Despite methodological limitations, another study has recently emphasized the crucial role of deep pressure touch for social bonding and potential clinical effects [20].

Standardized observer and self-rating scales for depression or the general state of well-being can and should be used to assess touch effects, although one should keep in mind that according to our own experience, patients after a potentially emotionally deeply "touching" massage might not feel extremely motivated to do a mass of paperwork. Visual analogue scales constructed individually on the basis of foregoing open trials and informal exchange with the patients about their reactions toward the applied treatment might often be the better choice to assess short-term effects [18,21]. Besides, there is the need to consider qualitative approaches in future research, e.g., by using (un)structured in-depth interviews aiming to gain insights into the subjective experience of patients and healthy volunteers. Although touch research has emphasized the psychological dimensions of affective touch by demonstrating positive effects on pleasantness and well-being assessed via standardized rating scales, there is a considerable lack of research elucidating the qualitative nature of these feelings in a differentiated manner. The preference for neuroscientific approaches over phenomenological research still dominates modern clinical psychiatry and may have limited the understanding of the subjective experiences that constitute the core of psychopathology [22]. Therefore, we argue for a consideration of phenomenological approaches that can be mixed with the quantitative paradigm to provide further insights into the "corporeality" [22] of mental disorders and the intervening function of touch therapies. A "qualitative turn" in touch research could also facilitate the generation of innovative hypotheses and might contribute to the development of a theory of human touch. From an epistemological point of view touch research should aim at not explaining the effects of touch in a purely reductionistic model being based on a single explanatory level and fostering a scientifically unsound mixing-up of psychological processes and brain functions. Instead, we argue for the exploration and discussion of the underlying mechanisms on separate explanatory levels.

A particularly tricky question in designing randomized-controlled trials in this scientific field is the choice of an adequate control condition. In view of the prevailing skepticism as to the usefulness of body-oriented treatments in psychiatric indications, it is essential to take care of a methodically conservative approach. Since "placebo controls" are difficult to be established, waiting lists or more or less boring "relax" videos have sometimes been used as controls that will provide the researcher with the prospect of more or less guaranteed positive effects of touch. Rapaport et al. recently presented a compelling research design that compared massage therapy with a light touch condition (laying on of hands) in patients with generalized anxiety disorders to identify effective touch techniques for managing clinical conditions [23]. The potential influences of, e.g., the appearance, age, sex (see, e.g., [24]) and empathy of the massage therapists and the special experimental environment should be reduced, e.g., by keeping the general experimental conditions as equal as possible in both groups. By giving special attention to this special methodical aspect, we might be able to isolate the effects of touch itself from other unspecific influences. There is a further need to establish equivalence studies comparing massage therapy's efficacy with traditional approaches or standard care. Naturalistic studies will also provide more insight into the effectiveness of touch therapies in general settings.

Several mechanisms of action have been discussed, which could explain massage therapy's clinical effects in patients suffering from affective disorders [16,25]. However, research to clarify these mechanisms is still in its infancy but could be conducive to the acceptance of touch therapies (see, e.g., [26]). The concept of interoception (i.e., "the sense of the physiological condition of the body" [27]) and its modification by various therapeutic approaches currently gains special attention. There is cumulative evidence for an association of various mental disorders with interoceptive impairments such as blunted heartbeat perception accuracy or maladaptive attention styles towards somatic feelings [28,29]. Interoceptive treatments are currently under development [30]; however, they focus mainly on mindfulness-based approaches [31], whose effectiveness in mental disorders may have been overestimated [32] and whose applicability to severely affected patients is limited [33,34]. Although affective touch offers an easy and safe access to the interoceptive system, the skin has so far received little attention as a modulator of interoceptive states. In a recent paper, we have proposed an interoceptive mechanism of action that could explain the well-documented anti-depressive effects of massage therapy by considering touch receptors in the skin that probably mediate the restoration of impaired interoceptive states [35]. To the best of our knowledge, this hypothesis has never been tested, although theoretical considerations support its fundamentals. Previous research has also validated instruments allowing the assessment of multidimensional self-reported interoception to identify interoceptive predictors of treatment outcome [36]. Moreover, another promising mechanism of massage therapy could be found in the promotion of restorative sleep patterns, which are probably associated with analgesic effects [37].

Touch may not be considered only as a therapeutic factor in psychiatry, since it also has a preventive function for mental health. This appears of particular importance in view of the detrimental effects of social isolation on morbidity and mortality in various cohorts [38]. An abundance of previous work has shown beneficial effects of gentle touch in the mother–infant dyad that have been identified as a resilience factor reducing the risk for later psychopathology and promoting attachment [39]. Baby massage has gained broad acceptance in many countries. However, only a small number of studies referred to the effects of massage on full-term newborns; stabilized sleep patterns, reduced bilirubin levels in jaundice and alleviating effects on maternal depression have been reported [40]. Evidence exists that depressed mothers give their babies less positive touch, which is likely to be compensated for by increased infant self-touching [41].

The applicability of affective touch in children as well as in elderly residents of nursing homes needs more attention and scientific approaches. Touch therapies and basal stimulation techniques could serve as a non-pharmacological strategy to deal with agitation in patients suffering from dementia [42]. Touch could also play a prominent role in patients who are cognitively unable to receive psychotherapy, such as individuals with severe intellectual disability [43]. As to psycho-oncology, some authors have contributed promising evidence on the supportive, analgesic, and relaxing effects of professional touch in cancer patients [44].

In summary, there is an urgent need for high-quality clinical trials examining and confirming the beneficial psychophysical effects of touch therapies in psychiatry. Further experimental research elucidating the mechanisms of action behind the mental effects of massage therapy certainly would also strengthen the acceptance of this intervention by public authorities, clinical medicine and the scientific community.

Conflicts of Interest: The authors declare no conflict of interest.

References

1. Galea, S.; Merchant, R.M.; Lurie, N. The Mental Health Consequences of COVID-19 and Physical Distancing. *JAMA Intern. Med.* **2020**, *180*, 817. [CrossRef] [PubMed]
2. McGlone, F.; Wessberg, J.; Olausson, H. Discriminative and affective touch: Sensing and feeling. *Neuron* **2014**, *82*, 737–755. [CrossRef] [PubMed]
3. Cascio, C.J.; Moore, D.; McGlone, F. Social touch and human development. *Dev. Cogn. Neurosci.* **2019**, *35*, 5–11. [CrossRef] [PubMed]
4. Seaman, L. Affective nursing touch. *Geriatr. Nurs.* **1982**, *3*, 163–164. [CrossRef]
5. Field, T. Massage therapy research review. *Complement. Ther. Clin. Pract.* **2016**, *24*, 19–31. [CrossRef]
6. Boehme, R.; van Ettinger-Veenstra, H.; Olausson, H.; Gerdle, B.; Nagi, S.S. Anhedonia to Gentle Touch in Fibromyalgia: Normal Sensory Processing but Abnormal Evaluation. *Brain Sci.* **2020**, *10*, 306. [CrossRef]
7. Cassileth, B.R.; Vickers, A.J. Massage therapy for symptom control: Outcome study at a major cancer center. *J. Pain Symptom Manag.* **2004**, *28*, 244–249. [CrossRef]
8. Cuijpers, P.; van Straten, A.; Bohlmeijer, E.; Hollon, S.D.; Andersson, G. The effects of psychotherapy for adult depression are overestimated: A meta-analysis of study quality and effect size. *Psychol. Med.* **2010**, *40*, 211–223. [CrossRef]
9. Kirsch, I.; Deacon, B.J.; Huedo-Medina, T.B.; Scoboria, A.; Moore, T.J.; Johnson, B.T. Initial severity and antidepressant benefits: A meta-analysis of data submitted to the Food and Drug Administration. *PLoS Med.* **2008**, *5*, e45. [CrossRef]
10. Hengartner, M.P.; Angst, J.; Rössler, W. Antidepressant Use Prospectively Relates to a Poorer Long-Term Outcome of Depression: Results from a Prospective Community Cohort Study over 30 Years. *Psychother. Psychosom.* **2018**, *87*, 181–183. [CrossRef]
11. Jakobsen, J.C.; Katakam, K.K.; Schou, A.; Hellmuth, S.G.; Stallknecht, S.E.; Leth-Møller, K.; Iversen, M.; Banke, M.B.; Petersen, I.J.; Klingenberg, S.L.; et al. Selective serotonin reuptake inhibitors versus placebo in patients with major depressive disorder. A systematic review with meta-analysis and Trial Sequential Analysis. *BMC Psychiatry* **2017**, *17*, 58. [CrossRef]
12. Van Dam, N.T.; van Vugt, M.K.; Vago, D.R.; Schmalzl, L.; Saron, C.D.; Olendzki, A.; Meissner, T.; Lazar, S.W.; Kerr, C.E.; Gorchov, J.; et al. Mind the Hype: A Critical Evaluation and Prescriptive Agenda for Research on Mindfulness and Meditation. *Perspect. Psychol. Sci.* **2018**, *13*, 36–61. [CrossRef] [PubMed]
13. Paykel, E.S.; Ramana, R.; Cooper, Z.; Hayhurst, H.; Kerr, J.; Barocka, A. Residual symptoms after partial remission: An important outcome in depression. *Psychol. Med.* **1995**, *25*, 1171–1180. [CrossRef] [PubMed]
14. Wu, P.; Fuller, C.; Liu, X.; Lee, H.-C.; Fan, B.; Hoven, C.W.; Mandell, D.; Wade, C.; Kronenberg, F. Use of complementary and alternative medicine among women with depression: Results of a national survey. *Psychiatr. Serv.* **2007**, *58*, 349–356. [CrossRef] [PubMed]
15. Baumgart, S.; Müller-Oerlinghausen, B.; Schendera, C.F.G. Efficacy of massage therapy on depression and anxious disorders as well as on depressiveness and anxiety as comorbidity—A systematic overview of controlled studies. *Phys. Med. Rehab. Kuror.* **2011**, *21*, 167–182. [CrossRef]
16. Moyer, C.A.; Rounds, J.; Hannum, J.W. A meta-analysis of massage therapy research. *Psychol. Bull.* **2004**, *130*, 3–18. [CrossRef]
17. Hou, W.-H.; Chiang, P.-T.; Hsu, T.-Y.; Chiu, S.-Y.; Yen, Y.-C. Treatment effects of massage therapy in depressed people: A meta-analysis. *J. Clin. Psychiatry* **2010**, *71*, 894–901. [CrossRef]
18. Arnold, M.M.; Müller-Oerlinghausen, B.; Hemrich, N.; Bönsch, D. Effects of Psychoactive Massage in Outpatients with Depressive Disorders: A Randomized Controlled Mixed-Methods Study. *Brain Sci.* **2020**, *10*, 676. [CrossRef]

19. Baumgart, S.B.-E.; Baumbach-Kraft, A.; Lorenz, J. Effect of Psycho-Regulatory Massage Therapy on Pain and Depression in Women with Chronic and/or Somatoform Back Pain: A Randomized Controlled Trial. *Brain Sci.* **2020**, *10*, 721. [CrossRef]
20. Case, L.K.; Liljencrantz, J.; McCall, M.V.; Bradson, M.; Necaise, A.; Tubbs, J.; Olausson, H.; Wang, B.; Bushnell, M.C. Pleasant Deep Pressure: Expanding the Social Touch Hypothesis. *Neuroscience* **2020**. [CrossRef]
21. Müller-Oerlinghausen, B.; Berg, C.; Scherer, P.; Mackert, A.; Moestl, H.-P.; Wolf, J. Effects of slow-stroke massage as complementary treatment of depressed hospitalized patients. Results of a controlled study (SeSeTra). *Dtsch. Med. Wochenschr.* **2004**, *129*, 1363–1368. [CrossRef] [PubMed]
22. Fuchs, T. Corporealized and disembodied minds: A phenomenological view of the body in melancholia and schizophrenia. *Philos. Psychiatr. Psychol.* **2005**, *12*, 95–107.
23. Rapaport, M.H.; Schettler, P.; Larson, E.R.; Edwards, S.A.; Dunlop, B.W.; Rakofsky, J.J.; Kinkead, B. Acute Swedish Massage Monotherapy Successfully Remediates Symptoms of Generalized Anxiety Disorder: A Proof-of-Concept, Randomized Controlled Study. *J. Clin. Psychiatry* **2016**, *77*, e883–e891. [CrossRef] [PubMed]
24. Reichert, B. Does the Therapist's Sex Affect the Psychological Effects of Sports Massage?-A Quasi-Experimental Study. *Brain Sci.* **2020**, *10*, 376. [CrossRef]
25. Rapaport, M.H.; Schettler, P.J.; Larson, E.R.; Carroll, D.; Sharenko, M.; Nettles, J.; Kinkead, B. Massage Therapy for Psychiatric Disorders. *Focus (Am. Psychiatr. Publ.)* **2018**, *16*, 24–31. [CrossRef]
26. Ribeiro-Blanchard, A.; Comfort, W.E. Keeping in Touch with Mental Health: The Orienting Reflex and Behavioral Outcomes from Calatonia. *Brain Sci.* **2020**, *10*, 182. [CrossRef]
27. Craig, A.D. How do you feel? Interoception: The sense of the physiological condition of the body. *Nat. Rev. Neurosci.* **2002**, *3*, 655–666. [CrossRef]
28. Eggart, M.; Lange, A.; Binser, M.J.; Queri, S.; Müller-Oerlinghausen, B. Major depressive disorder is associated with impaired interoceptive accuracy: A systematic review. *Brain Sci.* **2019**, *9*, 131. [CrossRef]
29. Khalsa, S.S.; Adolphs, R.; Cameron, O.G.; Critchley, H.D.; Davenport, P.W.; Feinstein, J.S.; Feusner, J.D.; Garfinkel, S.N.; Lane, R.D.; Mehling, W.E.; et al. Interoception and Mental Health: A Roadmap. *Biol. Psychiatry Cogn. Neurosci. Neuroimaging* **2018**, *3*, 501–513. [CrossRef]
30. Farb, N.; Daubenmier, J.; Price, C.J.; Gard, T.; Kerr, C.; Dunn, B.D.; Klein, A.C.; Paulus, M.P.; Mehling, W.E. Interoception, contemplative practice, and health. *Front. Psychol.* **2015**, *6*, 763. [CrossRef]
31. Khoury, N.M.; Lutz, J.; Schuman-Olivier, Z. Interoception in Psychiatric Disorders: A Review of Randomized, Controlled Trials with Interoception-Based Interventions. *Harv. Rev. Psychiatry* **2018**, *26*, 250–263. [CrossRef]
32. Coronado-Montoya, S.; Levis, A.W.; Kwakkenbos, L.; Steele, R.J.; Turner, E.H.; Thombs, B.D. Reporting of Positive Results in Randomized Controlled Trials of Mindfulness-Based Mental Health Interventions. *PLoS ONE* **2016**, *11*, e0153220. [CrossRef] [PubMed]
33. Dobkin, P.L.; Irving, J.A.; Amar, S. For Whom May Participation in a Mindfulness-Based Stress Reduction Program be Contraindicated? *Mindfulness* **2012**, *3*, 44–50. [CrossRef]
34. Hanssen, I.; van der Horst, N.; Boele, M.; van Lochmann Bennekom, M.; Regeer, E.; Speckens, A. The feasibility of mindfulness-based cognitive therapy for people with bipolar disorder: A qualitative study. *Int. J. Bipolar Disord.* **2020**, *8*, 33. [CrossRef] [PubMed]
35. Eggart, M.; Queri, S.; Müller-Oerlinghausen, B. Are the antidepressive effects of massage therapy mediated by restoration of impaired interoceptive functioning? A novel hypothetical mechanism. *Med. Hypotheses* **2019**, *128*, 28–32. [CrossRef] [PubMed]
36. Eggart, M.; Valdés-Stauber, J. Can changes in multidimensional self-reported interoception be considered as outcome predictors in severely depressed patients? A moderation and mediation analysis. Advance online publication. *J. Psychosom. Res.* **2020**. [CrossRef]
37. Sunshine, W.; Field, T.M.; Quintino, O.; Fierro, K.; Kuhn, C.; Burman, I.; Schanberg, S. Fibromyalgia benefits from massage therapy and transcutaneous electrical stimulation. *J. Clin. Rheumatol.* **1996**, *2*, 18–22. [CrossRef]
38. Holt-Lunstad, J.; Smith, T.B.; Layton, J.B. Social relationships and mortality risk: A meta-analytic review. *PLoS Med.* **2010**, *7*, e1000316. [CrossRef]
39. Norholt, H. Revisiting the roots of attachment: A review of the biological and psychological effects of maternal skin-to-skin contact and carrying of full-term infants. *Infant Behav. Dev.* **2020**, *60*, 101441. [CrossRef]
40. Cleveland, L.; Hill, C.M.; Pulse, W.S.; DiCioccio, H.C.; Field, T.; White-Traut, R. Systematic Review of Skin-to-Skin Care for Full-Term, Healthy Newborns. *J. Obstet. Gynecol. Neonatal Nurs.* **2017**, *46*, 857–869. [CrossRef]
41. Herrera, E.; Reissland, N.; Shepherd, J. Maternal touch and maternal child-directed speech: Effects of depressed mood in the postnatal period. *J. Affect. Disord.* **2004**, *81*, 29–39. [CrossRef] [PubMed]
42. Margenfeld, F.; Klocke, C.; Joos, S. Manual massage for persons living with dementia: A systematic review and meta-analysis. *Int. J. Nurs. Stud.* **2019**, *96*, 132–142. [CrossRef] [PubMed]
43. Chan, J.S.-L.; Tse, S.H.-M. Massage as therapy for persons with intellectual disabilities: A review of the literature. *J. Intellect. Disabil.* **2011**, *15*, 47–62. [CrossRef] [PubMed]
44. Boyd, C.; Crawford, C.; Paat, C.F.; Price, A.; Xenakis, L.; Zhang, W. The Impact of Massage Therapy on Function in Pain Populations-A Systematic Review and Meta-Analysis of Randomized Controlled Trials: Part II, Cancer Pain Populations. *Pain Med.* **2016**, *17*, 1553–1568. [CrossRef] [PubMed]

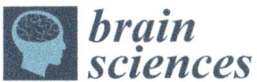

Article

Effects of Psychoactive Massage in Outpatients with Depressive Disorders: A Randomized Controlled Mixed-Methods Study

Michaela Maria Arnold [1,2,*], Bruno Müller-Oerlinghausen [3], Norbert Hemrich [2] and Dominikus Bönsch [1,4]

1. Medizinische Fakultät, Julius-Maximilians-Universität Würzburg, 97070 Würzburg, Germany; dominikus.boensch@bezirkskrankenhaus-lohr.de
2. Berufsfachschule für Massage am Universitätsklinikum Würzburg, 97080 Würzburg, Germany; Hemrich_N@ukw.de
3. Charité, Universitätsmedizin Berlin, 10117 Berlin, Germany; bruno.mueller-oerlinghausen@web.de
4. Bezirkskrankenhaus für Psychiatrie, Psychotherapie und Psychosomatische Medizin, 97816 Lohr am Main, Germany
* Correspondence: michaela-maria-arnold@web.de

Received: 9 August 2020; Accepted: 21 September 2020; Published: 26 September 2020

Abstract: The clinical picture of depressive disorders is characterized by a plethora of somatic symptoms, psychomotor retardation, and, particularly, anhedonia. The number of patients with residual symptoms or treatment resistance is high. Touch is the basic communication among humans and animals. Its application professionally in the form of, e.g., psychoactive massage therapy, has been shown in the past to reduce the somatic and mental symptoms of depression and anxiety. Here, we investigated the effects of a specially developed affect-regulating massage therapy (ARMT) vs. individual treatment with a standardized relaxation procedure, progressive muscle relaxation (PMR), in 57 outpatients with depression. Patients were given one ARMT or PMR session weekly over 4 weeks. Changes in somatic and cognitive symptoms were assessed by standard psychiatric instruments (Hamilton Depression Scale (HAMD) and the Bech–Rafaelsen–Melancholia–Scale (BRMS)) as well as a visual analogue scale. Furthermore, oral statements from all participants were obtained in semi-structured interviews. The findings show clear and statistically significant superiority of ARMT over PMR. The results might be interpreted within various models. The concept of interoception, as well as the principles of body psychotherapy and phenomenological aspects, offers cues for understanding the mechanisms involved. Within a neurobiological context, the significance of C-tactile afferents activated by special touch techniques and humoral changes such as increased oxytocin levels open additional ways of interpreting our findings.

Keywords: massage therapy; psychoactive massage; affect-regulating massage therapy; affective touch; depression; pain; interoception; C-tactile fibers; body psychotherapy

1. Introduction

Depressive disorders are among the most common mental diseases in the western world [1]. In addition to the personal suffering of those affected and their environment, the disease represents a significant challenge for society as a whole. Lifetime prevalence has been found to range between 16% and 20%. The World Health Organization (WHO) has declared that it will become the leading cause of global disease burden in the future [2]. The course of the disorder in most patients is episodic and is characterized by a lowered, depressed mood lasting for at least 2 weeks, vital and cognitive retardation, negative thoughts, and the core symptom of anhedonia inflicting nearly all areas of normal life and making life dull and gray. Suicidal ideation and suicidal behavior occur frequently; 10–15% of patients with affective disorders who do not receive efficacious prophylactic long-term treatment (e.g., with lithium salts) will finally die from suicide. In addition, a plethora of somatic symptoms, including pain and physical fatigue affect quality of life, impair working function, increase healthcare utilization, worsen depression outcomes, and increase the risk of recurrence [3]. There is further evidence that depression is associated with substantially disturbed body awareness and desynchronization causing psychomotor retardation [4,5]. These aspects do not receive sufficient consideration if depression is simply called a "mood disorder" or "affective disorder" [6].

It is important to realize that the body ("Leib" in German language and philosophy) of a depressed individual is affected just as much as the mental state. Many facets of colloquial language illustrate the close connection of body and depression, e.g., talking about a person who is depressed or mortified, we may say "he/she is down in the mouth".

Although the diagnosis and treatment of depression has improved significantly in recent years, there are still deficits in the care and therapy of affected individuals. Optimal treatment success often cannot be achieved, so that in about 30% of cases residual symptoms can be observed. These include primarily, sleep disorders, chronic depressed and/or anxious mood, cognitive deficits, and somatic symptoms [7,8].

The main treatment modalities comprise different types of psychotherapy and/or treatment with antidepressants and other psychotropic agents. However, although prescriptions for antidepressants are rising from year to year in most European countries and in the US [9], their overall efficacy is far from satisfactory. In recent years critical voices based on meta-analyses and serious, independent studies have drawn the attention of a larger audience to the fact that in some patient cohorts the therapeutic efficacy of antidepressants was not found to be higher than that of placebo [10–12]. On the other side, increased awareness of patients, doctors, and the general public has been directed particularly to adverse reactions to these compounds, such as a worsened course of the illness, increased cardiovascular mortality, suicidal ideation, or persistent sexual disturbances even after withdrawal [13,14]. Furthermore, it also appears that the beneficial effects of psychotherapy on depression were overestimated in the past [15]. This might be the reason why patients with depression often seek help and relief from their symptoms with "alternative" or complementary therapies [16].

Treatment strategies such as body-oriented methods, including mindfulness-based approaches, have been discussed and explored recently, e.g., body psychotherapy for the management of chronic depression [17]. There is also sufficient evidence for the effectiveness of, e.g., physical training such as aerobic exercise for depression [18,19]. In addition, elements from yoga, tai chi, and qigong are increasingly being investigated and used to treat mental disorders, but evidence of their efficacy is preliminary [20,21].

Survey data suggest frequent utilization of massage therapy or other hands-on treatment among patients with depression [16]. Whether a passive treatment modality such as massage therapy would have a beneficial effect on symptoms of depression presents an intriguing question in view of the great number of patients with treatment-resistant depression [22] and the practical lack of side effects of most types of massage [23]. In medical practice, positive effects of massage therapy, such as relaxation or anxiety relief, and antidepressant effects have been observed. These clinical experiences are supported by a meta-analysis of available studies. On the basis of 10 randomized controlled trials (RCTs) comprising 249 participants, Moyer et al. (2004) found that treatment resulted in a lower post-treatment level of depression than in 73% of the control subjects. The authors considered this finding as persuasive evidence for an antidepressive effect in particular and concluded that the medium effect size equaled that of psychotherapy [24]. In addition, they also found strong evidence for reduced trait anxiety. An earlier meta-analysis by Peters (1999), however, had concluded that existing studies on the effectiveness of massage as a nursing intervention had only limited validity and that more rigorous research would be needed [25]. A meta-analysis of 17 RCTs was performed by Hou et al. in 2010, indicating significant effectiveness in the treatment vs. control groups in spite of only moderate quality of the included studies [26]. Baumgart et al. (2011) presented findings from a systematic survey of 22 carefully selected randomized studies published between 1996 and 2009, including seven studies on patients with depression, anxiety, or exhaustion/fatigue as the main diagnosis [27]. All seven studies, only two of them on hospitalized patients, showed a significant reduction in anxiety symptoms, and depression was significantly reduced in five studies. However, the authors also underlined that the heterogeneity of the diagnoses and the diversity of the controls and the assessment methods still limited valid general conclusions on the efficacy of massage therapy in the treatment of depression.

The website of the American Massage Therapy Association (www.amtamassage.org) clearly documents the still existing paucity of controlled studies in this area and the need for further studies recruiting patients with clinical depression. There is a great variety of massage methods, such as Swedish massage, Esalen massage, Thai massage, etc. [28–30]. Our research group has been concentrating for many years on studying the clinical effects of affective touch, also called soft or gentle touch or psychoactive massage, in patients and healthy volunteers. In a previous randomized controlled trial, the application of a specially developed one-hour psychoactive massage (Slow Stroke®Massage) showed antidepressive efficacy in hospitalized patients with depression [31]. Sufficient evidence could be provided that within the special setting of this study, gentle touch was the key element to produce the antidepressive/anxiolytic effect on the behavioral and somatic level. In the present study, we investigated the mental and subjective somatic effects of a special form of psychoactive massage, the affect-regulating massage therapy (ARMT) vs. progressive muscle relaxation (PMR) in outpatients with depression. (PMR has become an established relaxation method over the last decades and is already used regularly in the psychiatric and psychosomatic field [32,33]). A direct comparison of the effectiveness of psychoactive massage therapy and PMR in patients with depression has not been done so far. The present study, therefore, tested the following hypotheses:

Hypothesis 1. *It is expected that the application of ARMT will prove to be more effective in positively influencing the behavioral and somatic dimensions related to depression than a standardized relaxation method such as PMR. This difference will be reflected in the observer ratings using the assessment instruments described below.*

Hypothesis 2. *It is expected that a stronger effect in favor of ARMT will also be seen in patients' self-assessments. Significant results are expected in the pre-post differences of at least half of the items tested on a specially developed visual analogue scale.*

2. Materials and Methods

2.1. Study Design

The study was designed as a two-arm, monocentric, randomized controlled intervention study with a fixed number of cases. Every patient in the intervention group received four weekly treatments by means of a standardized massage technique (ARMT). Patients in the control group received four applications of PMR over the same time period. Before starting and immediately after completing the study, patients were assessed by an external rater blinded to the specific treatments the patients had been assigned to. A visual analogue scale was used for self-assessment, which was filled in by the patients before and after each treatment. The study center was the outpatient clinic of the vocational school for massage at the University Hospital of Würzburg (Würzburg, Germany), directed by N. Hemrich.

2.2. Instruments for Assessing Mental and Somatic Symptoms

2.2.1. HAMD

The Hamilton Depression Scale (HAMD) was used as the external assessment instrument [34,35]. A total of 17 items concerning the depressive symptoms of the previous seven days are checked. Each item is scored from 0 to 4. The severity of the depression is classified as follows [36]: 0–8 points:

no depression or clinically unremarkable or remitted; 9–16 points: mild depression; 17–24 points: moderate depression and ≥25 points: severe depression.

2.2.2. BRMS

The Bech–Rafaelsen Melancholia Scale (BRMS) was used as a further questionnaire for external assessment at multiple time points [37]. It comprises a total of 11 items, which refer to the depressive symptoms of the previous three days. Each item is scored between 0 and 4. The interrater reliability of the German version has been found to be $r = 0.80$ and higher [38]; it has also generally been found to be $r = 0.80$ and higher. The severity of depression is classified according to the sum of all scores as follows: 0–5 points: no depression; 6–14 points: mild depression; 15–25 points: moderate depression and 26–44 points: severe depression.

2.2.3. VAS

A specially designed 100 mm visual analogue scale (VAS) was used for subjective assessment of depressive symptoms consisting of 8 items for self-assessment of the current mood [39]. It was completed by the patients immediately before and after each intervention in order to document changes that occurred during the intervention. Only the symptom of sleep disorder could not be recorded due to the given time frame. In addition, patients could write down free-form personal comments. The following items, indicating the negative poles (zero points) of the scale, were assessed:

VAS 1: Stress/tension
  "I'm very tense"/"I'm completely relaxed"
VAS 2: Hopelessness
  "I feel hopeless"/"I'm full of hope"
VAS 3: Internal unrest
  "I am very restless"/"I am full of inner peace"
VAS 4: Pain sensations
  "I'm feeling pain"/"I'm not feeling any pain"
VAS 5: Psychomotor retardation
  "I feel rigid and immobile"/"I feel light and lively"
VAS 6: Tendency to brood
  "Negative thoughts are circulating in my head"/"I'm thinking positive and optimistic"
VAS 7: Loss of drive
  "I feel limp and listless"/"I feel full of energy and drive"
VAS 8: Unpleasant physical sensations
  "I'm not comfortable in my body"/"I'm comfortable in my body"

2.2.4. Assessment on Clinical Interview

The initial examination included an assessment of the patient's general history as well as a detailed disease-focused interview. After the end of the treatment series, a final consultation was held. During this semi-structured interview, the patient's subjective experiences and attitudes toward the study were questioned and documented. All interviews were conducted by the principal investigator (first author) and recorded in writing.

2.3. Conducting the Study

2.3.1. Sample Size Calculation

The study by Müller-Oerlinghausen et al. served as the basis for the sample size calculation [31,40]. The mean values and mean differences between pre- and post-assessments and the standard deviation could be derived with regard to VAS. Differences of about 20 scale points with a standard deviation of

25 had been described for several VAS variables. Against this empirical background and assuming a significance level of 5% for two-sided tests, we calculated an optimal sample size of 58.75 cases, which was rounded up to 60. No potential attrition rate was taken into consideration.

2.3.2. Ethical Approval

The study was approved by the Ethics Committee of the Medical Faculty of the Julius Maximilian University of Würzburg. Performance of the study, including informed consent of the patients, followed the Declaration of Helsinki.

2.3.3. Recruitment and Randomization

The patients were recruited in cooperating psychiatric or psychotherapeutic practices in Würzburg. Advertisements were placed in the press and leaflets were distributed at the University Hospital of Würzburg.

Inclusion criteria were as follows:

- Patients of both sexes between the ages of 18 and 65;
- The presence of a mild to moderate depressive episode diagnosed by a general practitioner or specialist, including the following ICD-10 diagnoses: F32.0, F32.1, F32.2, F32.8, F32.9, F33.0, F33.1, F33.2, F33.8, F33.9.

Exclusion criteria:

- Acute comorbid medical condition.
- Eczematous skin disease;
- Marked varicose veins or venous thrombosis;
- Pregnancy;
- Simultaneous participation in another clinical trial.

The first contact of potential study participants was usually made by phone or email. Suitability for participation in the study was checked on the basis of the inclusion and exclusion criteria. If there was agreement, the patient's written consent to participate in the study was then obtained. Within two months, 60 patients were recruited. Randomization took place in the order of admission to the study. A randomization list was used, which was based on numbers from the random number generator of the SPSS® statistical program package. After being notified of the randomization result, three participants in the control group terminated their participation in the study prematurely because they did not agree with the assigned group. This resulted in 30 participants in the intervention group and 27 participants in the control group. The initial rating was carried out by an external observer blinded with regard to the randomization result. The threshold for inclusion in the study was set before as 9 points on the HAMD 17 and 6 points on the BRMS. No financial or other compensation was offered to the study participants. The process is shown in Figure 1.

2.4. Description of Interventions (ARMT and PMR)

2.4.1. Massage Group (ARMT)

The study was performed in cooperation with the vocational school for massage at the University Hospital of Würzburg. A working group was formed consisting of nine masseurs under training, the principal of the vocational school, and the principal investigator/first author, who is also a certified massage therapist. Through intensive training and communication, a standardized treatment procedure was developed, which was carried out by all therapists equally. Techniques for psychoactive massage described in the literature, e.g., Slow Stroke© Massage [28,31], were taken as the matrix for developing our own massage technique, described in detail below. (To get an idea of these special touch techniques ref. also to some video material under www.bruno-mueller-oerlinghausen.de or www.affective-touch.com).

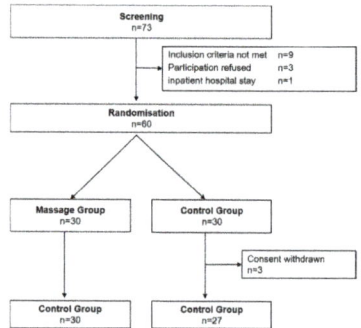

Figure 1. Recruitment and randomization.

Any massage session lasted 60 min including rest. It took place in a quiet room. A constant room temperature of at least 25 °C was ensured. The massage oil was preheated to 35 °C. Massage always began with the undressed patient in a supine position. The genital area was covered by a towel. At the beginning, the preheated massage oil was distributed on the ventral body surface to the abdomen, legs, and arms to ensure continuous treatment without interruption. Afterwards, the therapist's hands rested on the palmar side of the patient's feet to achieve conscious contact. Subsequently, extensive whole-body strokes were performed. Both hands were used to massage from the legs over the flanks up to the arms and over the pelvis and legs, and back to the starting point. This was followed by treatment of the lower extremities with superficial, partially stretching strokes and soft kneading. The sequence was continued by strokes from the middle of the body cranially and caudally as a diagonal whole-body stroke. After classical abdominal, thoracic, and arm treatment, as well as symmetrical whole-body strokes, the patient changed to the prone position. The treatment then began analogous to the ventral side, starting from the heel bone and continuing over the legs, back, and arms. This was followed by a sequence of diagonal and symmetrical whole-body strokes and soft kneading of the dorsal body. Finally, to mark the end of the treatment, the hands rested on the plantar sides of the feet. The patient was then allowed to rest for another 10–15 min. During this time, he or she was covered with sheets and a woolen blanket. Overall, the treatment was carried out very calmly and evenly. Possible muscular tension was not addressed in order to not interrupt the massage flow by any painful perceptions. No conversations were held during the treatment and no background music was played. Care was taken to ensure that patients were always treated by the same therapist within a treatment series.

2.4.2. Control Group (PMR)

In the control group, progressive muscle relaxation (PMR) according to Jacobson, a widely recognized relaxation method, was used [32,33]. In order to make the general conditions as equivalent as possible to those of the massage group, PMR was not performed in the group, but as an individual 45-min treatment. The instructions were given by the same therapists who were also active in the massage group. At the beginning of PMR, the patient was asked to get into in a comfortable supine position, using a massage table or gymnastics mat as a base. Care was taken to ensure a comfortable position through appropriate room temperature and the use of pillows and blankets. The patient was then individually guided through a PMR whole-body schedule. The standardized instructions were presented in a calm and pleasant tone. Afterwards, the patient could rest for 10–15 min. During the treatment, no conversations were held and no background music was played. Care was taken to ensure that the patients were always treated by the same therapist within one series.

2.5. Accompanying Therapy

Any existing therapy with psychotropic drugs and/or psychotherapy could be continued. Changes in this respect were documented at the end of the trial period.

2.6. Statistical Evaluation

Absolute and relative frequencies, as well as mean and standard deviation, were used to present personal data such as age, gender, marital status, etc. All data collected manually by the questionnaire were first transferred to an Excel spreadsheet. Data were then analyzed using IBM SPSS Statistics (version 25). Since normal distribution of the parameters could not be assumed, the Mann–Whitney U-test, a nonparametric test, was chosen to calculate statistical significance. The level of statistical significance was set as $p < 0.05$ (two-sided). Pearson's correlation coefficient r was calculated for estimation of effect size.

3. Results

3.1. Description of Sample

3.1.1. Sociodemographic Data

The ARMT group consisted of 30 participants. The mean age was 45.2 years; the youngest patient was 24, the oldest, 60 years old; 76.7% were female. About half of the participants were married or in a stable partnership (53.3%). The majority of participants (76.7%) had an intermediate or high school diploma and had qualified employment.

The PMR group consisted of 27 participants. The mean age was 45.0 years; the youngest patient was 19, the oldest, 64 years old; 81.5% of were female. About half of the participants were married or living in a stable partnership (55.6%). Almost all participants (96.3%) had an intermediate or high school diploma and had qualified employment; in this respect they were somewhat different from the subjects of the ARMT group. The sociodemographic data is shown in Table 1.

Table 1. Sociodemographic variables of the two patient groups.

	ARMT	$n = 30$	PMR	$n = 27$
	M	SD	M	SD
Age (years)	45.2	9.43	44.9	12.29
Sex	n	%	n	%
female (n)	22	73.33	22	81.48
male (n)	8	26.67	5	18.52
Civil status				
single	9	30.00	9	33.33
married/partnership	16	53.33	15	55.55
divorced/widowed	5	16.67	3	11.11
Children				
childless	11	36.67	15	55.55
one or two children	13	43.33	6	22.22
three or more children	6	20.00	6	22.22
Education				
primary school	7	23.33	1	3.7
secondary school	13	43.33	25	92.6
high school	10	33.33	1	3.7
Employment				
vocational training	23	76.67	22	81.48
academic career	7	23.33	5	18.52
unemployed	6	20.00	7	25.92

ARMT = affect regulating massage therapy; PMR = progressive muscle relaxation; M = Mean; SD = Standard Deviation.

3.1.2. Depression-Related Data

In the ARMT group, the severity of depression was rated as moderately severe, corresponding to 18.2 points on average on the HAMD at the beginning of the study. Assessment by means of the BRMS (mean value 16.1 points) also confirmed moderately severe depression. Psychopharmacological treatment as mono- or combination therapy was reported by 56.7% of the participants. There was no change in dosage for 83.3% of the patients over the duration of the study. About half (53.33%) of the participants were under psychotherapeutic treatment during participation in the study.

In the PMR group, the severity of depression rated by means of the HAMD averaged 19.2 points at the beginning of the study, also indicating a moderately severe depressive episode. The BRMS scores suggested an identical classification, with an average of 17.4 points. Psychopharmacological treatment as mono or combination therapy accounted for 55.5% of the participants. There was no change in dosage for 85.2% of the participants during participation in the study. Almost half (48.2%) of the participants were under psychotherapeutic treatment during the study.

3.2. Effects of ARMT and PMR Assessed by HAMD and BRMS

The averaged differences between the HAMD assessment at time TA, before the first treatment, and time TB, after the fourth treatment, were calculated. The reduction in symptom burden over 4 weeks was significantly more pronounced in the ARMT group than in the control group ($p = 0.034$, $r = 0.28$). The results are shown in Figure 2.

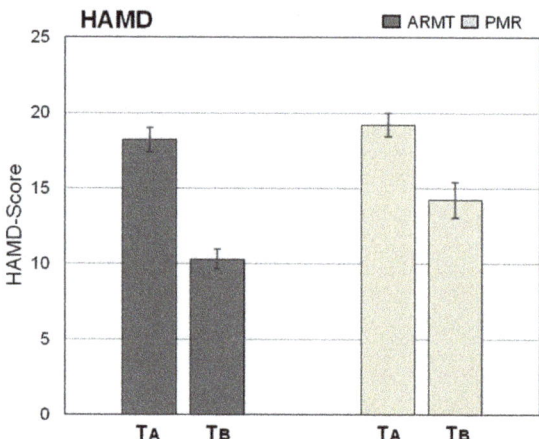

Figure 2. Summed up Hamilton Depression Scale (HAMD) scores in ARMT and PMR groups before (TA) and after (TB) completing the full series of treatments (mean ± SEM).

Focusing on individual items of the HAMD, changes in the following items proved to be highly statistically significant with a moderate effect size:

- HAMD 1: Depressive mood ($p = 0.004$, $r = 0.39$)
- HAMD 13: Somatic symptoms ($p = 0.021$, $r = 0.30$)

Although statistical significance was not reached, we consider the numerical change of item five (sleep disorders) to be particularly noteworthy ($p = 0.059$, $r = 0.25$). The course of the BRMS scores is depicted in Figure 3. The reduction in symptom burden during 4 weeks was significantly more pronounced in the massage group than in the control group ($p = 0.04$, $r = 0.27$). Focusing on individual items, the difference of the following single BRMS dimensions over time proved to be statistically significant:

- BRMS 8: Emotional retardation ($p = 0.037$, $r = 0.28$)
- BRMS 9: Sleep disorders ($p = 0.038$, $r = 0.28$)

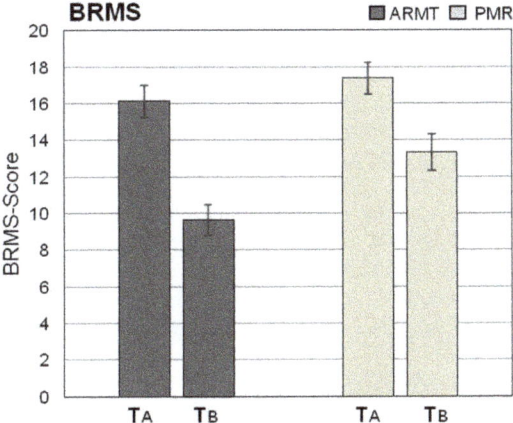

Figure 3. Summed up Bech–Rafaelsen Melancholia Scale (BRMS) scores in ARMT and PMR groups before (TA) and after (TB) completing the full series of treatments (mean ± SEM).

Although statistical significance was not achieved, special attention might be given to the change in item one, motor activity ($p = 0.063$, $r = 0.25$).

In summary, the findings so far are in accordance with Hypothesis 1 (see above).

3.3. Results of Participant's Self-Assessment (VAS)

For each VAS item (one to eight), the pre-post differences related to each treatment session were averaged over time points T1–T4. Figure 4 shows that the treatment effects were markedly and significantly more pronounced in the ARMT group as compared to the PMR group. Statistical significance of this difference existed for six of the eight items. (Descriptions of single items can be found in Section 2.2.3).

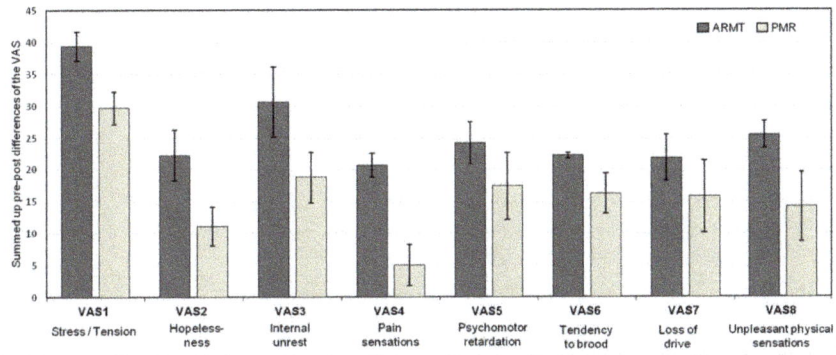

Figure 4. Averaged differences (± SD) of individual pre-/post-treatment visual analogue scale (VAS) values over total study period (T1–T4).

Please note that a value of 100 on, e.g., VAS 1 ("tension") would signify that the proband felt completely relaxed. (A score of 100 is always the positive pole and zero the negative pole of each

VAS item.) In detail, the following individual VAS items show (highly) significant changes in favor of the massage treatment, i.e., greater pre-post differences of particularly those variables closely associated with depression:

VAS 1: Stress/tension ($p = 0.035$, $r = 0.28$)
VAS 2: Hopelessness ($p = 0.032$, $r = 0.28$)
VAS 3: Internal unrest ($p = 0.009$, $r = 0.35$)
VAS 4: Pain sensations ($p = 0.003$, $r = 0.39$)
VAS 5: Psychomotor retardation ($p = 0.012$, $r = 0.33$)
VAS 8: Unpleasant physical sensations ($p = 0.011$, $r = 0.34$)

A moderate effect size was observed for most of the changes. The pre-post differences in VAS 6 (tendency to brood/negative thoughts, $p = 0.075$, $r = 0.24$) and VAS 7 (lack of drive, $p = 0.070$, $r = 0.24$) were not different between the two treatment groups. To illustrate the therapeutic process, Figure 5, as an example, presents the time course of VAS 5, psychomotor retardation (pre- and post-treatment scores) over the four treatment sessions. Obviously, the treatment effects are more marked in the ARMT group.

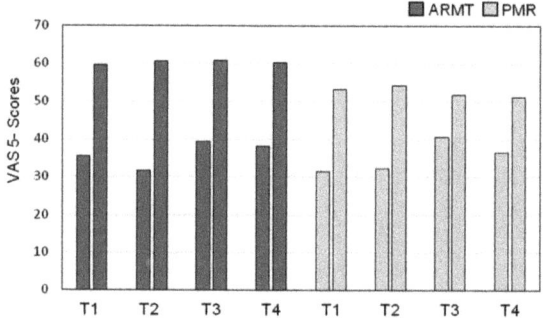

Figure 5. Time course of VAS 5 (psychomotor retardation) scores over time points $T1$–$T4$ in ARMT vs. PMR groups. Arithmetic means before and after treatment (right and left columns, respectively). Note: A score of 100 signifies that the proband agrees fully with the statement "My body feels light and mobile".

Consequently, Hypothesis 2 could be confirmed, i.e., it is expected that a stronger effect will also be seen in the patients' self-assessment. Significant results are assumed in at least half of the VAS items.

3.4. Statements of Study Participants in Clinical Interviews

The statistical results are underlined by the personal statements of the study participants. Particularly frequent positive comments were made by patients assigned to the massage group:

- Better body awareness and deep relaxation;
- Interruption of brooding and negative thoughts;
- Increased motivation for everyday life activities.

As points of criticism, some patients mentioned a feeling of coldness and a sense of shame about taking off their clothes before the massage.

Additionally, patients in the control group described positive effects of PMR:

- Useful in everyday life and as a sleeping aid;
- Easy relaxation and better body awareness.

The lack of background music was occasionally mentioned as a point of criticism. Patients in both groups indicated that they had particularly benefited from the morning sessions. The early treatment appointment significantly reduced the burden of a matutinal depressive mood and had a positive effect for the rest of the day. Some participants also experienced a continuous increase in the perceived positive effects during the course of the study. As a point of criticism, study participants from both groups mentioned particular unfavorable external conditions, such as noise from the adjacent construction site.

4. Discussion

As outlined above, somatic symptoms such as psychomotor retardation, sleep disorders, or general fatigue are prominent features of the clinical picture of depression. Thomas Fuchs perceives depression as a physical illness existing not only against the background of functional disorders of the entire organism, such as dysregulation of the hormone system and biorhythmics, metabolic and immunological changes. Rather, as a phenomenologist, he describes a disorder of the basic physical constitution that presents itself as a "corporisation of the body" (ref. [41] the contrasting significance of "corpse" and "body" in English). Like an objectification, the patient experiences himself distanced from his body-self and no longer "at home in his body", as the sociologist Hartmut Rosa illustrates it in general terms. The depressed person does not feel "comfortable in his skin", where the skin in Rosa's terminology constitutes an organ of resonance [42]. This disturbed bodily feeling manifests itself in different regions, such as tightness in the chest, heaviness of the limbs, or chronic fatigue. The body loses drive and spontaneity. Everything feels heavy. This is also reflected in the subject's exchange with the environment: breathing is flattened, facial expressions are reduced, libido is often tuned down. The "feeling of numbness" overshadows every perception, so that even crying is no longer possible. It is not mourning that is felt, but the feeling of emptiness and lifelessness that is expressed primarily in the body. "Being a body is replaced by having a body" [43]. Would it not be possible that the cognitive and emotional characteristics of depression are secondary reactions to the perception of the primary bodily changes [44,45]?

Hartmut Rosa tries to separate the depressive experience from grief: "Grief is an element of a relationship to the world that is, on the whole, quite resonant. [. . .] Depression, on the other hand, is characterized by the fact that there are no more tears: the relationship to the world can no longer be liquefied, it is petrified" [42]. The patient feels unable to counteract this weighing feeling of heaviness, and this fundamental phenomenon might induce speculation on a potential bridge to the concept of "learned helplessness" [46].

Against this background, it seems a rational approach to use body-oriented therapies in the treatment of depression. Our findings indicate antidepressive, anxiolytic, and analgesic effects, which were significantly more pronounced among the participants in the massage therapy group as compared to those in the PRM group. How can these remarkable therapeutic effects of a professional, empathetic, affective touch technique be explained? We shall discuss some options on various explanatory levels.

One of the most obvious effects of massage therapy, according to the patients' self-assessment, is the pronounced psychomotor relaxation, which is also reflected in the reduction in inner restlessness. However, it was not only general tension that was released by the treatment. Rather, feelings of hopelessness and inner restlessness were also significantly reduced. The therapeutic touch technique also had a positive effect on the existing obsessive brooding tendency. In the final open talks with the patients, we often heard statements such as that the massage finally allowed the individual to "turn off my thoughts" or "to break loose". One patient made a written comment after the third massage session: "Never before did I experience such a deep relaxation. None of the usual relaxing (mind–body) exercises had this strong effect".

However, even if this feeling of relaxation is a significant part of the overall effect, there must be other factors involved, otherwise the superiority of massage over a standardized relaxation method would hardly make sense. In modern theories of depression, the concept of interoception has been given increasing attention [47,48]. Interoception, i.e., the perception of the processes of the body's interior, distinguishes between proprioception (perception of body position and movement in space) and visceroception (perception of the inner organs' activity). In contrast to exteroception, the signals making up interoception are sent from the entire inner milieu of the individual to the brain. Interoception can likewise be understood as a skill that can be trained through regular practice (e.g., in mindfulness methods), thus contributing to a more conscious body perception and better emotional self-regulation.

In order to explain the effects of the body-oriented interventions examined in this study, we may refer to this concept. The external conditions per se that were more or less concordant in both groups provided a framework for increased body perception. A calm atmosphere without distractions was created to enable the patients to experience consciously their bodily condition, in the sense of an "inner view". The special feature of affective touch is the calm, mindful approach enabling patients to consciously experience their body. This procedure can thus be described as an intensive training of interoception. The patients' oral statements underline this assumption.

Recently a hypothesis was put forward that the antidepressive effect of affective touch can be explained by a normalization of disturbed interoception [49]. Another special factor that could explain the significant superiority of affect-regulating massage based on its basic element, affective touch, is the factor of touch itself. A gentle, empathetic touch is generally experienced as pleasant. It can soothe feelings of social exclusion and facilitate interpersonal binding [50,51]. The neurophysiological correlates of this type of touch have been intensively investigated during the last two decades. The specific feeling of well-being that humans and hairy mammals experience with this type of touch is based neurophysiologically on the activation of so-called C-actile afferents. In particular, Swedish researchers were able to show that a neuronal network of slowly conducting, non-myelinated C-fibers reacts to special receptors of the hairy skin (located, e.g., on the back of the hand, but not on the palm). For these receptors, gentle, slow, and rhythmic touch at a speed of about 3 cm/sec is the appropriate stimulus, projected directly and predominantly into the insular area. The stimulation of such C tactile fibers seems to have as its only "purpose" creating a feeling of well-being [52]. This might also have evolutionary biological significance, e.g., by promoting the feeling of kinship within a group. Other afferent projections via A-beta or A-alpha fibers as well as signals from mechanoreceptors in the hairy skin most likely will also contribute to the overall interoceptive signaling taking place in various limbic structures.

Switching to the level of experience and behavior, it should be kept in mind that touch is the basal medium of communication among humans and animals [53,54]. Against the background of anhedonia, described as the most common feature of depressive experience and behavior, our findings are in some way "paradoxical". How can patients with depression feel and express bodily and verbally affective touch as a positive experience? Obviously empathic, professional touch can slip into this basic communication disorder, i.e., can enter the disturbed emotional world of the patient. It fits into this concept that participants in the massage group often expressed feelings of having been "accepted" in the final talks with the first author. The following English translation of a patient's original final statement might help us in understanding some essentials of the therapeutic process:

"I cried a lot the first time. For the first time I was able to feel my legs and my feet. Tears of joy during the treatment. From the second session onwards, even better with a warming pad. Meeting of the hands on my belly—very touching. I never experienced such a loving touch before. With further treatments I was loosening up completely. Already during the second session I perceived more than the first time. Even my hands were treated! Because of the depression I couldn't allow touching me otherwise.... My shell has become softer, my heart is opened. The massage therapist was totally super gentle, helped me to become a "whole person" again".

Even though the patient quoted above was in all probability not familiar with the work of Wilhelm Reich [55], in her description she nevertheless takes up an essential aspect that plays an important role in modern body psychotherapy [56]. In Reichian terminology, one can speak of an armoring of the emotions [55], which can be influenced, if not eliminated, by massage therapy. According to our observations, patients often are taken by surprise that after a massage session their body feels "less heavy". A trusting therapist–patient relationship in the field of physiotherapy seems to be just as important as is already recognized in psychotherapy. The therapeutic relationship thrives on appropriate empathy and the right balance between affectionate empathy and professional demarcation. In contrast to psychotherapy, however, in the physiotherapeutic context it is specifically the body of the patient that is perceived and accepted and thus enters into resonance with the therapist. This leads to new, possibly corrective (body) experiences, which can be of decisive importance for the therapeutic process. To quote the clinical psychologist C.A. Moyer from his meta-analysis of studies on the effects of massage therapy in depression: "The finding that massage therapy has an effect on trait anxiety and depression that is similar in magnitude to what would be expected to result from psychotherapy suggests the possibility that these different treatments may be more similar than previously considered" [24].

However, coming back to the mechanism involved, a decisive difference exists in healing touch: according to Changaris, we offer the patient direct affect-regulating "bottom-up" therapy in contrast or addition to the "top-down" technique of cognitive psychotherapy [57]. Finally, humoral effects such as increased oxytocin levels and reduced cortisol, e.g., in saliva might add to the interpretation of the antidepressive effects of psychoactive massage within a neurobiological context [58,59]. Oxytocin has been attributed with significant effects on social interaction, as well as feelings of trust and connectedness [60]. Thus, it does not seem unlikely that depressive patients suffering from social withdrawal and isolation could profit from increased oxytocin release, possibly facilitating contact and communication [61]. Additionally, the analgesic effects of massage therapy might be related to increased oxytocin release [62]. Tiffany Field [58], against the background of various experimental studies, has often emphasized the importance of markedly reduced cortisol levels in urine or saliva of various diagnostic groups of depressed or stressed patients having been given massage therapy. The strong relaxing effect observed also in our patients might well be related to this hormonal change. Tiffany Field, however, has often argued that the lowered cortisol levels are related to increased vagal activity [63].

4.1. Strengths of the Study

4.1.1. Control Group

It was already pointed out that the choice of an adequate control group, besides the impossibility of blinding, is one of the biggest methodical problems in developing a meaningful design in massage studies. Often the control conditions are chosen in such a way that only a standard therapy, waiting list, or general relaxation (quiet sitting/lying, relaxing music or movies) is used. In our study, a more adequate procedure was chosen instead, which led to the most equal conditions possible for all study participants, with the essential difference that therapeutic touch occurred only in the massage group. This allowed us to strengthen the evidence that it is not a bunch of mostly unknown unspecific effects such as personal devotion, but the affective touch as such that is responsible for the greater effectiveness of massage therapy. "Adequate control conditions" signifies that participants in both the massage and control groups always received individual treatments. PMR is typically performed as group therapy. It can be assumed that performing PMR as an individual treatment increased its effectiveness. In other words, we selected a rather conservative approach, which resulted in moderate effect sizes. Use of a "placebo" control would most likely produce much greater effect sizes. In addition, an identical group of therapists were involved in both groups in order to avoid distorting personal influence. Furthermore, the same premises were used for both the massage and control groups. All treatments took place in comparable periods within four months and in a constant environment.

4.1.2. Study Participants

Relatively few studies on the efficacy of massage therapy have been conducted so far in patients with mental illness. The present study provides further evidence of the positive effects of massage therapy in depression. In selecting the study participants, we focused on patients with mild to moderate depression whose clinical picture and disease severity reflected a broad section of the general population. In this way we were able to create largely realistic conditions as they are encountered daily in practices of both GPs and psychiatrists, but also physiotherapists.

4.1.3. Assessments

Standardized and widely used psychiatric scales for assessing and quantifying depressive symptoms were employed in validated German translation.

4.1.4. Conducting the Study

In both groups, care was taken to ensure the consistency of therapists in individual treatment series. In addition to reducing variance, this also served to maximize the effects, as other studies have shown the importance of therapist consistency [64]. Furthermore, all therapists were equally prepared for the study owing to intensive training. This ensured a standardized and comparable execution of individual therapies.

4.2. Limitation

One important criterion for the quality of studies contributing to the bulk of evidence-based medicine, besides randomization and active control, is the blinding of study participants and directly involved investigators. For obvious methodological reasons, this requirement could not be met in the present study, as in many comparable studies. However, according to a recent meta-analysis, the absolute postulate of blinding when carrying out a sound study might be somewhat questioned in the future [65]. Furthermore, the self-assessment questionnaires (before and after each treatment) were handed out to the patients by the treating therapists themselves. In retrospect, the critical question came up as to whether this circumstance may have led to distortion. One may speculate whether it would have been important for some patients to leave a positive impression or not to "disappoint" the therapist by filling out a questionnaire in a neutral or negative way. However, since the same questionnaire handling was used in both groups, this possible bias was not further discussed, which might have caused a greater overall effect, but probably did not distort the difference between the two groups

4.3. Outlook

Due to the limited effectiveness of the currently available and widely used treatments in depression, it seems reasonable to expand the therapeutic spectrum for inpatients and outpatients with body-oriented procedures. In this context, affect-regulating or comparable psychoactive massage therapies represent a noteworthy opportunity to open up new access routes for acute treatment. They can be used as low-threshold offerings in the outpatient setting in order to achieve a rapid antidepressive effect. Their use in an inpatient setting is also conceivable according to the findings of a previous controlled study [31]. Very good adherence can be expected, as the present study was also able to prove. Body-oriented therapeutic approaches should be given higher value within the spectrum of antidepressive treatments. They also deserve a special place beside much propagated mind–body techniques [66,67]. A severely depressed patient will often be unable to participate in special psychological training sessions aimed at stress reduction.

5. Conclusions

This randomized controlled intervention study examined the psychophysical effects of body-oriented treatment methods on patients suffering from mild to moderate depression in an outpatient setting. We tested the hypothesis that a one-hour massage based on a special gentle touch technique (affect regulating massage therapy = ARMT) is superior in its positive effects to a relaxation method that has long been established in the clinical field, progressive muscle relaxation according to Jacobson. Our results confirm this assumption. In both the observer ratings and self-assessments of patients using a visual analogue scale, statistically significant superiority of massage therapy was shown. When focusing on individual dimensions of the HAMD, the superior effects were particularly evident in the items "depressive mood" and "general somatic symptoms". Assessment using the BRMS showed statistically significant superiority of massage therapy particularly in the items "emotional retardation" and "sleep disorders". As for the sleep disorders so often encountered in patients with depression, it should be noted that massage had a positive effect, especially on difficulty remaining asleep, while difficulty getting to sleep responded better to PMR. This observation also coincides with the free-form statements of some study participants who used the PMR technique outside of the study, independently as an aid to fall asleep. Especially in the self-assessment (VAS) of patients, massage therapy proved to be superior. This became obvious for the vast majority of items questioned. When inspecting the pre-post differences of individual VAS items, the stronger impact of massage therapy on the dimensions stress/tension, internal unrest, unpleasant physical sensation, psychomotor retardation, and hopelessness is particularly impressive. Changes were also marked for pain sensations. Overall, we were able to document the doubtless superiority of ARMT for core symptoms of depressive experience and behavior.

Author Contributions: M.M.A.: conceptualization, investigation, writing—review and editing; B.M.-O.: methodology, supervision, writing—original draft; N.H.: resources; D.B.: supervision. All authors have read and agreed to the published version of the manuscript.

Funding: This research received no external funding. The publication is supported by the "open access program" of Julius-Maximilians-Universität, Wuerzburg, Germany.

Acknowledgments: Thanks are due to Ulrich Stefenelli for his advice and help in statistical matters and to Michael Eggart for methodical input. Thanks are also due the Karl and Veronica Carstens Foundation (Essen, Germany) for scientific advice during M.M.A.'s work on her doctoral thesis.

Conflicts of Interest: The authors declare no conflict of interest.

References

1. Jacobi, F.; Höfler, M.; Strehle, J.; Mack, S.; Gerschler, A.; Scholl, L.; Busch, M.A.; Maske, U.; Hapke, U.; Gaebel, W.; et al. Psychische Störungen in der Allgemeinbevölkerung: Studie zur Gesundheit Erwachsener in Deutschland und ihr Zusatzmodul Psychische Gesundheit (DEGS1-MH). *Nervenarzt* **2014**, *85*, 77–87. [CrossRef] [PubMed]
2. *Depression and Other Common Mental Disorders: Global Health Estimates*; World Health Organization: Geneva, Switzerland, 2017.
3. Kapfhammer, H.P. Somatic symptoms in depression. *Dial. Clin. Neurosci.* **2006**, *8*, 227–239.
4. Fuchs, T.; Schlimme, J.E. Embodiment and psychopathology: A phenomenological perspective. *Curr. Opin. Psychiatry* **2009**, *22*, 570–575. [CrossRef] [PubMed]
5. Fuchs, T. Melancholia as a desynchronization. Towards a psychopathology of interpersonal time. *Psychopathology* **2001**, *34*, 179–186. [CrossRef]
6. Danielsson, L.; Rosberg, S. Depression embodied: An ambigous striving against fading. *Nord. Coll. Caring Sci.* **2014**, *29*, 501–509. [CrossRef]
7. Paykel, E.S.; Ramana, R.; Cooper, Z.; Hayhurst, H.; Kerr, J.; Barocka, A. Residual symptoms after partial remission: An important outcome in depression. *Psychol. Med.* **1995**, *25*, 1171–1180. [CrossRef]
8. Nierenberg, A.A. Residual symptoms in depression: Prevalence and impact. *J. Clin. Psychiatry* **2015**, *76*, e1480. [CrossRef]
9. Lohse, M.; Müller-Oerlinghausen, B. Psychopharmaka. In *Arzneiverordnungsreport 2019*; Schwabe, U., Paffrath, D., Ludwig, W.-D., Klauber, J., Eds.; Springer: Berlin, Germany, 2019; pp. 927–959.
10. Cuijpers, P.; Cristea, A. What if a placebo effect explained all the activity of depression treatments? *World Psychiatry* **2015**, *14*, 310–311. [CrossRef]

11. Munkholm, K.; Paludan-Müller, A.S.; Boesen, K. Considering the methodological limitations in the evidence base of antidepressants for depression: A reanalysis of a network meta-analysis. *BMJ Open* **2019**, *9*, e024886. [CrossRef]
12. Pigott, H.E.; Leventhal, A.M.; Alter, G.S.; Boven, J.J. Efficacy and effectiveness of antidepressants: Current status of research. *Psychother. Psychosom.* **2010**, *79*, 267–279. [CrossRef]
13. Fava, G.A.; Tomba, E.; Grandi, S. The road to recovery from depression. Don't drive today with yesterday's map. *Psychother. Psychosom.* **2007**, *6*, 260–265. [CrossRef] [PubMed]
14. Andrews, P.W.; Thomson, J.A.; Amstadter, A.; Neale, M.C. Primum nil nocere: An evolutionary analysis of whether antidepressants do more harm than good. *Front. Psychol.* **2012**, *3*, 117. [CrossRef] [PubMed]
15. Cuijpers, P.; van Straten, A.; Bohlmeijer, E. The effects of psychotherapy for adult depression are overestimated: A meta-analysis of study quality and effect size. *Psychol. Med.* **2010**, *40*, 211–223. [CrossRef] [PubMed]
16. Wu, P.; Fuller, C.; Liu, X.; Lee, H.; Fan, B.; Hoven, C.W.; Mandell, D.; Wade, C.; Kronenberg, F. Use of complementary and alternative medicine among women with depression: Results of a national survey. *Psychiatr. Serv.* **2007**, *58*, 349–356. [CrossRef]
17. Röhricht, F.; Papadopoulos, N.; Priebe, S. An exploratory randomized controlled trial of body psychotherapy for patients with chronic depression. *J. Affect. Dis.* **2013**, *151*, 85–91. [CrossRef]
18. Cooney, G.M.; Dwan, K.; Greig, C.A.; Lawlor, D.A.; Rimer, J.; Waugh, F.R.; McMurdo, M.; Mead, G.E. Exercise for depression. *Cochrane Database Syst. Rev.* **2013**, CD004366. [CrossRef]
19. Kvam, S.; Kleppe, C.L.; Nordhus, I.H.; Hovland, A. Exercise as a treatment for depression: A meta-analysis. *J. Affect. Disord.* **2016**, *202*, 67–86. [CrossRef]
20. Cramer, H.; Lauche, R.; Langhorst, J.; Dobos, G. Yoga for depression: A systematic review and meta-analysis. *Depress Anxiety* **2013**, *30*, 1068–1083. [CrossRef]
21. Oh, B.; Choi, S.M.; Inamori, A.; Rosenthal, D.; Yeung, A. Effects of qigong on depression: A systemic review. *Evid. Based Complement. Alternat. Med.* **2013**, *2013*, 134737. [CrossRef]
22. Jaffe, D.H.; Rive, B.; Denee, T.R. The humanistic and economic burden of treatment-resistant depression in Europe: A cross-sectional study. *BMC Psychiatry* **2019**, *19*, 247. [CrossRef]
23. Ernst, E. The safety of massage therapy. *Rheumatology* **2003**, *42*, 1101–1106. Available online: https://academic.oup.com/rheumatology/article/42/9/1101/1772218 (accessed on 2 May 2020). [CrossRef] [PubMed]
24. Moyer, C.A.; Rounds, J.; Hannum, J.W. A meta-analysis of massage therapy research. *Psychol. Bull.* **2004**, *130*, 3–18. [CrossRef] [PubMed]
25. Peters, R.H. The effectiveness of therapeutic touch: A meta-analytic view. *Nurs. Sci. Q.* **1999**, *12*, 52–61. [CrossRef] [PubMed]
26. Hou, W.H.; Chiang, P.T.; Hsu, Y.T.; Chiu, S.; Yen, Y.C. Treatment effects of massage therapy in depressed p2eople: A meta-analysis. *J. Clin. Psychiatry* **2010**, *71*, 894–901. [CrossRef] [PubMed]
27. Baumgart, S.; Müller-Oerlinghausen, B.; Schendera, C.F.G. Efficacy of massage therapy on depression and anxious disorders as well as on depressiveness and anxiety as comorbidity. A systematic overview of controlled studies. (Article in German with English abstract). *Phys. Rehab. Kur. Med.* **2011**, *21*, 167–182. [CrossRef]
28. Reichert, B. (Ed.) *Massage-Therapie*; Georg Thieme: Stuttgart, Germany, 2015.
29. Hoyme, R.J. *The Complete Guide to Modern Massage: Step-by-Step Massage Basis and Techniques from Around the World*; Althea Press: New York, NY, USA, 2018.
30. Müller-Oerlinghausen, B.; Kiebgis, G.M. *Berührung- Warum Wir Sie Brauchen und Wie Sie Uns Heilt*, 2nd ed.; Ullstein: München, Germany, 2018.
31. Müller-Oerlinghausen, B.; Berg, C.; Scherer, P.; Mackert, A.; Moestl, H.P.; Wolf, J. Effects of slow-stroke massage as complimentary treatment of depressed hospitalized patients: Results of a controlled study (SeSeTra). (Article in German with English abstract). *Dtsch. Med. Wochenschr.* **2004**, *129*, 1363–1368.
32. Jacobson, E. *Entspannung als Therapie: Progressive Relaxation in Theorie und Praxis*, 7th ed.; Klett-Cotta: Stuttgart, Germany, 2011.
33. Petermann, F. *Entspannungsverfahren: Das Praxishandbuch. Mit E-Book Inside*; Neuausgabe, 6., überarbeitete Auflage; Julius Beltz GmbH & Co: Weinheim, Germany, 2020.
34. Hamilton, M. A rating scale for depression. *J. Neurol. Neurosurg. Psychiatry* **1960**, *23*, 56–62. [CrossRef]
35. Weyer, G.; Koeppen, D. *Internationale Skalen für Psychiatrie 6*; überarb. und erw. Aufl; Beltz-Test: Göttingen, Germany, 2015.

36. Zimmerman, M.; Martinez, J.H.; Young, D.; Chelminski, I.; Dalrymple, K. Severity classification on the Hamilton Depression Rating Scale. *J. Affect. Disord.* **2013**, *150*, 384–388. [CrossRef]
37. Stieglitz, R.D. *Bech-Rafaelsen-Melancholie-Skala*; Hogrefe: Göttingen, Germany, 1998.
38. Maier, W.; Philipp, W. Comparative analysis of observer rating scales. *Acta Psychiatr. Scand.* **1985**, *72*, 239–245. [CrossRef]
39. Schomacher, J. Gütekriterien der visuellen Analogskala zur Schmerzbewertung. *Physioscience* **2008**, *4*, 125–133. [CrossRef]
40. Müller-Oerlinghausen, B.; Berg, C.; Droll, W. Die Slow Stroke Massage als ein körpertherapeutischer Ansatz bei Depression. *Psychiatr. Prax.* **2007**, *34*, S305–S308. [CrossRef] [PubMed]
41. Fuchs, T. Corporealized and disembodied minds. A phenomenological view of the body in melancholia and schizophrenia. *Psychiatry Psychol.* **2005**, *12*, 95–107.
42. Rosa, H. *Resonanz: Eine Soziologie der Weltbeziehung*, 1st ed.; Suhrkamp: Berlin, Germany, 2016.
43. Faller, H. *Depression: Klinik, Ursachen, Therapie*; Königshausen & Neumann: Würzburg, Germany, 2011.
44. Röhricht, F. Leibgedächtnis und Körper-Ich: Zwei zentrale Bezugspunkte in der störungsspezifischen körperorientierten Psychotherapie. *Psychol. Österreich.* **2011**, *4*, 239–248.
45. Gallagher, S. *How the Body Shapes the Mind*; Oxford University Press: New York, NY, USA, 2005.
46. Seligman, M.E.P. Learned helpnessless. *Ann. Rev. Med.* **1972**, *23*, 407–412. [CrossRef] [PubMed]
47. Eggart, M.; Lange, A.; Binser, M.J.; Queri, S.; Müller-Oerlinghausen, B. Major Depressive disorder is associated with Impaired interoceptive accuracy: A systematic review. *Brain Sci.* **2019**, *9*, 131. [CrossRef] [PubMed]
48. Arikha, N. The Interoceptive Turn. The Science of How We Sense Ourselves from within, Including Our Bodily States, is Creating a Radical Picture of Selfhood. 2019. Available online: https://aeon.co/essays/the-interoceptive-turn-is-maturing-as-a-rich-science-of-selfhood (accessed on 9 June 2020).
49. Eggart, M.; Queri, S.; Müller-Oerlinghausen, B. Are the antidepressive effects of massage therapy mediated by restoration of impaired interoceptive functioning? A novel hypothetical mechanism. *Med. Hypotheses* **2019**, *128*, 28–32. [CrossRef]
50. Von Mohr, M.; Kirsch, L.P.; Fotopoulou, A. The soothing function of touch: Affective touch reduces feelings of social exclusion. *NeuroImage* **2018**, *169*, 162–171. [CrossRef]
51. Takeuchi, M.S.; Miyaoka, H.; Tomoda, A.; Suzuki, M.; Liu, Q.; Kitamura, T. The effect of interpersonal touch during childhood on adult attachment and depression: A neglected area of family and developmental psychology? *J. Child Fam. Stud.* **2010**, *19*, 109–117. [CrossRef]
52. Olausson, H.; Wessberg, J.; Morrison, I.; McGlone, F. *Affective Touch and the Neurophysiology of CT Afferents*; Springer: New York, NY, USA, 2016.
53. Montagu, A. *Touching: The Human Significance of the Skin*; Columbia University Press: New York, NY, USA; London, UK, 1971.
54. Field, T. Massage therapy research review. *Complement. Ther. Clin. Pract.* **2016**, *24*, 19–31. [CrossRef]
55. Reich, W. *Character Analysis*, 3rd ed.; Farrar, Straus, Giroux: New York, NY, USA, 1972.
56. Röhricht, F. Body oriented psychotherapy—The state of the art in empirical research and evidence based practice: A clinical perspective. *Body Mov. Dance* **2009**, *4*, 135–156. [CrossRef]
57. Changaris, M. *Touch: The Neurobiology of Health, Healing, and Human Connection*; LifeRhythm: Mendocino, CA, USA, 2015.
58. Field, T.; Hernandez-Reif, M.; Diego, M.; Schanberg, S.; Kuhn, C. Cortisol decreases and serotonin and dopamine increase following massage therapy. *Int. J. Neurosci.* **2005**, *115*, 1397–1413. Available online: https://www.tandfonline.com/doi/pdf/10.1080/00207450590956459?needAccess=true (accessed on 2 May 2020). [CrossRef] [PubMed]
59. Kosfeld, M.; Heinrichs, M.; Zak, P.J.; Fischbacher, U.; Fehr, E. Oxytocin increases trust in humans. *Nature* **2005**, *435*, 673–676. [CrossRef] [PubMed]
60. Uvnäs-Moberg, K. *The Hormone of Closeness: The Role of Oxytocin in Relationships1. Aufl*; Springer Spektrum: Berlin/Heidelberg, Germany, 2016.
61. Wang, J.; Lloyd-Evans, B.; Giacco, D.; Forsyth, R.; Nebo, C.; Mann, F.; Johnson, S. Social isolation in mental health: A conceptual and methodological review. *Soc. Psychiatry Psychiatr. Epidemiol.* **2017**, *52*, 1451–1461. [CrossRef] [PubMed]

62. Paloyelis, Y.; Krahé, C.; Maltezos, S.; Williams, S.C.; Howard, M.A.; Fotopoulou, A. The Analgesic Effect of Oxytocin in Humans: A Double-Blind, Placebo-Controlled Cross-Over Study Using Laser-Evoked Potentials. *J. Neuroendocrinol.* **2016**, *28*. [CrossRef] [PubMed]
63. Diego, M.A.; Field, T.; Hernandez-Reif, M. Vagal Activity, Gastric Motility, and Weight Gain in Massaged Preterm Neonates. *J. Pediatrics* **2005**, *147*, 50–55. [CrossRef] [PubMed]
64. Listing, M.; Reißhauer, A.; Krohn, M.; Voigt, B.; Tjahono, G.; Becker, J.; Klapp, B.F.; Rauchfuß, M. Massage therapy reduces physical discomfort and improves mood disturbances in women with breast cancer. *Psycho-Oncology* **2009**, *18*, 1290–1299. [CrossRef]
65. Moustgard, H.; Clayton, G.L.; Jones, H.E.; Boutron, I. Impact of blinding on estimated treatment effects in randomized clinical trials: Meta-epidemiological study. *BMJ* **2020**, *368*, 6802. [CrossRef]
66. Dorsett, M.D.; Friccione, G.L.; Benson, H. A new era for mind-body medicine. *N. Engl. J. Med.* **2020**, *382*, 1390–1391. [CrossRef]
67. Michalak, J.; Burg, J.; Heidenreich, T. Don't forget your body: Mindfulness embodiment and the treatment of depression. *Mindfulness* **2012**, *3*, 190–199. [CrossRef]

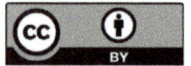

© 2020 by the authors. Licensee MDPI, Basel, Switzerland. This article is an open access article distributed under the terms and conditions of the Creative Commons Attribution (CC BY) license (http://creativecommons.org/licenses/by/4.0/).

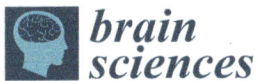

Article

Anhedonia to Gentle Touch in Fibromyalgia: Normal Sensory Processing but Abnormal Evaluation

Rebecca Boehme [1,2,*], Helene van Ettinger-Veenstra [2,3], Håkan Olausson [1,2,4], Björn Gerdle [2,3] and Saad S. Nagi [1,4]

1. Center for Social and Affective Neuroscience, Linköping University, 58185 Linköping, Sweden; hakan.olausson@liu.se (H.O.); saad.nagi@liu.se (S.S.N.)
2. Center for Medical Image Science and Visualization (CMIV), 58185 Linköping, Sweden; helenevanettinger@gmail.com (H.v.E.-V.); bjorn.gerdle@liu.se (B.G.)
3. Pain and Rehabilitation Centre, and Department of Health, Medicine and Caring Sciences, Linköping University, 58185 Linköping, Sweden
4. Department of Clinical Neurophysiology, Linköping University, 58185 Linköping, Sweden
* Correspondence: Rebecca.bohme@liu.se

Received: 30 March 2020; Accepted: 14 May 2020; Published: 18 May 2020

Abstract: Social touch is important for interpersonal interaction. Gentle touch and slow brushing are typically perceived as pleasant, the degree of pleasantness is linked to the activity of the C-tactile (CT) fibers, a class of unmyelinated nerves in the skin. The inability to experience pleasure in general is called anhedonia, a common phenomenon in the chronic pain condition fibromyalgia. Here, we studied the perception and cortical processing of gentle touch in a well-characterized cohort of fibromyalgia. Patients and controls participated in functional brain imaging while receiving tactile stimuli (brushing) on the forearm. They were asked to provide ratings of pleasantness of the tactile stimulus and ongoing pain. We found high distress, pain catastrophizing, and insomnia, and a low perceived state of health in fibromyalgia. Further, patients rated both slow (CT-optimal) and fast (CT-suboptimal) brushing as less pleasant than healthy participants. While there was no difference in brain activity during touch, patients showed deactivation in the right posterior insula (contralateral to the stimulated arm) during pleasantness rating and activation during pain rating. The opposite pattern was observed in healthy participants. Voxel-based morphometry analysis revealed reduced grey matter density in patients, in the bilateral hippocampus and anterior insula. Our results suggest anhedonia to gentle touch in fibromyalgia with intact early-stage sensory processing but dysfunctional evaluative processing. These findings contribute to our understanding of the mechanisms underlying anhedonia in fibromyalgia.

Keywords: touch; pain; C-tactile afferents; fibromyalgia; anhedonia; fMRI; posterior insula

1. Introduction

Fibromyalgia (FM) is a common, debilitating chronic pain condition. According to the American College of Rheumatology 1990 Criteria for the Classification of Fibromyalgia [1], the cardinal features comprise widespread pain and hypersensitivity, i.e., pain evoked by non-painful stimuli and exaggerated pain to painful stimuli. FM includes a myriad of other symptoms, including fatigue, sleep, and affective disturbances (e.g., anxiety and depression). The prevalence of FM is higher among females [2].

Social touch is important for human behavior and communication between individuals [3]. Pleasantness (or pleasure) associated with skin-to-skin contact is linked to a class of nerves in the skin, called C-tactile (CT) fibers. This is of considerable interest for questions about physical and social well-being and the interoceptive system [3]. CTs exhibit a unique 'inverted U-shaped' response pattern to brushing velocities, with slow brushing (1–10 cm/s, 'CT-optimal') producing a robust discharge—a stimulus that is perceived as pleasant and preferred by participants over fast brushing [4]. CTs have also been implicated in pain processing either directly or indirectly, as an allodynic substrate itself or through malfunctioning of this network [5,6].

While unmyelinated nociceptors have been the focus of earlier studies on fibromyalgia [7], less is known about the role of their low-threshold counterparts, the CTs. We have previously shown a blunted affective distinction between slow CT-optimal and fast CT-suboptimal brushing in FM patients, compared to healthy participants [8], suggesting a reduced CT input or processing in FM.

CT-optimal touch produces robust activation of the posterior insula with a somatotopic organization similar to that reported for cutaneous and muscle pain in healthy participants [9,10]. FM patients show higher activity in the insular cortex in response to painful stimuli (5), and have higher levels of glutamate in the posterior insula, an excitatory neurotransmitter associated with clinical pain and mechanical hypersensitivity in FM [11].

In the current study, we hypothesized to find differences in neural processing in the insular cortex, in response to CT-optimal touch in FM. In a group of well-characterized FM patients, we used fMRI to examine the cortical responses to slow and fast brush stroking and compared with matched healthy controls. In parallel, ratings for touch pleasantness and ongoing pain were collected. Grey matter density was also measured.

2. Materials and Methods

2.1. Participants

Female patients with a clinical diagnosis of FM, ranging between 25–55 years old, were recruited through the Pain and Rehabilitation Center at the Linköping University Hospital. These patients were recruited as part of a broader characterization of FM. Age- and gender-matched healthy controls (HC) were recruited through advertisements at the Linköping University and the University Hospital, and in the local news media. The Linköping Regional Ethics Review Board approved the study (Dnr 2016/471-32) and written informed consent was obtained after participants had read the complete study description, in accordance with the Declaration of Helsinki.

On the first visit, all participants underwent a clinical examination. To confirm the patients' eligibility, the eighteen tender points according to the FM classification criteria of the American College of Rheumatology [1] were clinically examined by senior consultants in rheumatology or pain medicine. This was performed in both patients and HC. Revised criteria for FM were recently presented [12,13], but these were not available in the finished form when the current study was designed and ethical approval was sought. The clinical examination also included registration of systolic and diastolic blood pressures. Weight (kg) and height (m) were also registered; body mass index (BMI; kg/m^2) was calculated as weight/height^2. At the time-point of the clinical examination, the subjects answered a health questionnaire covering demographic data as well as pain and psychological characteristics.

Exclusion criteria were MRI-incompatibility (claustrophobia or metal in the body), pregnancy, difficulty understanding Swedish, metabolic disease, neurological disease or severe psychiatric conditions, malignancy, rheumatoid arthritis, unregulated thyroid disease, cardiovascular disease, or lung disease. Another exclusion criterion was the inability to refrain from analgesics, including NSAIDs and sleep medication, for 48 h prior to the fMRI visit (i.e., a 48-h pharmacological washout period). Participants in the HC group reported having no current pain.

Functional imaging data of good quality were obtained for 31 patients (mean age, 39.0 ± 11.4 years) and 29 matched controls (mean age 42.7 ± 10.1 years).

2.2. Background Data

Age and gender were registered. FM patients also reported the duration of their condition in years.

2.2.1. Pain Intensity Aspects

A numeric rating scale (NRS) with anchor points 0 (denoting no pain) and 10 (denoting the worst imaginable pain) was used to capture the current pain (denoted by 'Pain Intensity Current') and the average pain intensity for the previous four weeks (denoted by 'Pain Intensity 4w').

2.2.2. Psychological Distress

The Hospital Anxiety and Depression Scale (HADS) was used to measure symptoms of anxiety and depression. The validated Swedish translation of HADS was chosen to reflect aspects of psychological distress [14,15] and had good psychometric characteristics [15,16]. HADS contains seven items in each of the depression and anxiety subscales (HAD-Depression and HAD-Anxiety). Both subscale scores ranged from 0–21. A score of 7 or less on each subscale was considered normal, a score of 8 to 10 indicated a possible abnormality, and a score of 11 or more indicated a definite abnormality [15]. In the present study, a score ≥ 11 was considered as having severe anxiety and depression symptoms.

2.2.3. Sleeping Problems

The Insomnia Severity Index (ISI) was used to quantify perceived insomnia severity. ISI captures the severity and impact of insomnia symptoms with good validity and internal consistency [17,18]. The seven items of ISI were rated on a five-point Likert scale (0–4). The scores of each item were added to calculate the total score of ISI (max = 28). The score could be divided into four categories–no insomnia (0–7), sub-threshold insomnia (8–14), moderate insomnia (15–21), and severe insomnia (22–28).

2.2.4. Pain Catastrophizing Scale (PCS)

PCS measures three dimensions of catastrophizing—rumination, magnification, and helplessness [19,20]—based on 13 items with anchor points ranging from 0 (not at all) to 4 (all the time). The current study used the total PCS (PCS-total); 52 was the maximum score according to the original scale and a high score represented a worse outcome. This instrument had good internal consistency, test-retest reliability, and validity [21].

2.2.5. Impact of the Pain Aspects

An NRS with anchor points 0 (denoted not at all) and 10 (denoted impossible to perform these activities) was used to capture to what extent the pain hindered daily activities (pain hindrance activities of daily living (ADL)), taking part in leisure activities including social and family activities (pain hindrance leisure), and working, including studies or homework (pain hindrance work). These items were only answered by the FM group.

2.2.6. The European Quality of Life Instrument (EQ-5D)

EQ-5D captured a patient's perceived state of health [22–24]. The first part of the instrument captured five dimensions—mobility, self-care, usual activities, pain/discomfort, and anxiety/depression. In the present study, we used the second part of the instrument and measured the current day's health on a 100-point scale, a thermometer-like scale (EQ-VAS) with defined endpoints (high values indicated good health and low values indicated bad health).

2.2.7. Pharmacological Treatments

Participants were asked to report their ongoing pharmacological treatments. Note that those included in the study were asked to refrain from analgesic use, including NSAIDs and sleep medication, for 48 h prior to the fMRI visit.

2.3. Stimuli and Procedures

2.3.1. Task

Before entering the MRI scanner, participants were instructed that they will be brushed on the forearm and were shown the rating scales. They were also brushed once on the forearm. During MRI, participants were brushed on the left forearm at two different velocities—3 cm/s (CT-optimal) and 30 cm/s (CT-suboptimal). The brusher, who was trained in the delivery of these stimuli, stood next to the scanner bore and received auditory cues over headphones. A 9-cm long line with 3-cm increments, was marked on the left forearm to aid the brusher to maintain the correct speed. The task consisted of three runs of 6 min each. In between runs, the participants were asked if they were alright in the scanner and okay to continue with the next run. In total, there were 15 repetitions of slow and fast brushing blocks, each lasting 12 s. The intertrial interval (ITI) between blocks was 10 to 12 s. The order of brushing velocities was randomized. During ITIs, participants looked at a fixation cross. Three times per condition (slow or fast), following a 10 to 12-s ITI, a question appeared on the screen asking the participant to rate the pleasantness of the brushing ("How pleasant is the stimulus?") and if they felt any pain ("Do you feel any pain?"). We formulated the latter question in this specific way because we assumed it might be difficult for the FM group to disentangle ongoing pain and specific pain related to the stimulus. This rating was therefore to be understood as rating of any ongoing pain. Using a button box in their right hand, participants moved a cursor on a visual analog scale (VAS) between the endpoints "unpleasant–pleasant" or "no pain–intense pain" (in Swedish). During analysis, the cursor positions were converted to their numerical values, ranging from −10 to +10 for pleasantness and 0 to 20 for pain. The pain ratings were not specifically related to brush-evoked sensation but to the subjects' general pain level.

2.3.2. MRI

Participants laid comfortably in a 3.0 Tesla Siemens scanner (Prisma, Siemens, Erlangen, Germany). Their left arm was placed on their belly and propped up by pillows. A 12-channel head coil was used to acquire 295 T2-weighted echo-planar images (EPI) per run, containing 48 multiband slices (TR = 1030 ms, TE = 30 ms, slice thickness = 3 mm, matrix size = 64 × 64, field of view = 488 × 488 mm, in-plane voxel resolution = 3 mm^2, flip angle = 63°). T1-weighted anatomical images were also acquired.

2.3.3. Analysis

Behavioral data were analyzed using SPSS (IBM Corp., Armonk, NY, USA). Ratings for slow and fast blocks were averaged. Ratings of the patient group were normally distributed; ratings of the control group were not due to a strong ceiling effect. Ratings were compared between conditions using paired t-test (FM) and Wilcoxon test (HC), and between groups, using Mann–Whitney U test. p-values < 0.05 were considered significant.

Functional MRI data were analyzed using statistical parametric mapping (SPM12, Wellcome Department of Imaging Neuroscience, London, UK; http://www.fil.ion.ucl.ac.uk/spm) in Matlab R2016a (The MathWorks, Natick, MA, USA). The following steps were performed—motion correction, co-registration of the mean EPI and the anatomical image, spatial normalization to the MNI T1 template, and segmentation of the T1 image, using the unified segmentation approach [25]. Normalization parameters were applied to all EPIs. All images were spatially smoothed with an isotropic Gaussian kernel of 6 mm full width, at half maximum. For statistical analysis of the BOLD response, the general linear model approach was used as implemented in SPM12. Using a block-design, the conditions (slow and fast) and the rating phase were convolved with the hemodynamic response function. Motion parameters were added as regressors of no interest. Family-wise-error (FWE) correction on the voxel level was used to correct for multiple comparisons on the whole-brain level and using small volume correction based on our a priori regions of interest (ROI). Based on previous studies [10,26], we were specifically interested in posterior insula activations, therefore, a posterior insula mask was used for small volume corrections (SVC) [27].

2.3.4. VBM

Voxel-based morphometry (VBM) was estimated using the VBM routine provided by the CAT12 toolbox (Gaser & Dahnke, Jena University Hospital, Departments of Psychiatry and Neurology) in SPM12. Total intracranial volume was included as a covariate. Groups were compared using a t-test at the whole brain level.

3. Results

3.1. Clinical Characteristics

The disease duration in the FM cohort was 4.4 years, on average, since diagnosis and as expected, they had a high number of tender points, i.e., at the group level, >16 out of 18. In HC, the tender points were scarcely found. FM patients had significantly higher blood pressure and BMI than HC. While HC reported no pain, both pain intensity measures (current and at 4 weeks) in FM patients were above 5 on the NRS. Distress, pain catastrophizing, and insomnia (HADS, PCS, and ISI) were significantly higher and overall health (EQ-VAS) was significantly lower in FM patients (Table 1).

Table 1. Age, pain characteristics, psychological variables, the impact of pain and health aspects in the fibromyalgia group (FM) and in the healthy controls (HC); mean and one standard deviation (SD).

Group	HC	$n = 29$	FM	$n = 31$	Statistics
Variables	Mean	SD	Mean	SD	p-Value
Age (years)	42.7	10.1	39.2	11.4	0.219
Systolic BP (mm Hg)	113.2	8.8	121.5	12.9	0.006
Diastolic BP (mm Hg)	75.3	8.5	80.6	10.6	0.040
Number of tender points	0.3	0.9	16.7	1.5	<0.001
FM duration (years)			4.4	5.0	NA
Height (m)	1.69	0.06	1.66	0.06	0.090
Weight (kg)	68.4	10.9	81.4	19.2	0.002
BMI (kg/m^2)	23.8	3.1	29.3	6.3	<0.001
Pain intensity current	0.0	0.0	5.7	1.8	<0.001
Pain intensity 4w	0.0	0.0	5.9	1.8	<0.001
HADS-Depression	1.4	1.7	6.0	3.6	<0.001
HADS-Anxiety	2.6	2.3	7.8	4.0	<0.001
PCS	11.8	9.2	20.3	10.5	0.001
ISI	4.5	4.5	13.4	5.9	<0.001
Pain hindrance ADL			5.7	2.3	NA
Pain hindrance leisure			5.7	2.5	NA
Pain hindrance work			4.9	2.7	NA
EQ-VAS	86.8	7.8	53.3	19.5	<0.001

BP = blood pressure; HADS = Hospital Anxiety and Depression Scale; PCS = Pain Catastrophizing Scale; ISI = Insomnia Severity Index; EQ-VAS = the health scale of EQ-5D (European Quality of Life instrument); w = weeks; NA = not applicable.

Four FM patients had more severe symptoms (≥11) according to the HADS-Depression subscale, compared to none in the HC. Corresponding figures for the HADS-Anxiety were eight patients in FM and none in HC. At least moderate insomnia (≥15) was found in 14 FM patients and in one HC.

Three FM patients and 26 HC did not use any pharmacological drugs. Those using medication among the FM cohort were often on several substances (range 1–5), including paracetamol ($n = 19$), antidepressant medication (selective serotonin reuptake inhibitor and serotonin-norepinephrine reuptake inhibitor, $n = 12$), tricyclic antidepressants ($n = 9$), opioids ($n = 7$), vitamins (e.g., B12, $n = 5$), medication for high blood pressure ($n = 3$), proton-pump inhibitors ($n = 3$), gabapentin ($n = 2$), antihistamine ($n = 2$), and other medications ($n = 9$). HC reported sumatriptan ($n = 1$), tricyclic antidepressant ($n = 1$), methotrexate ($n = 1$), and metoprolol ($n = 1$). All participants refrained from analgesics including NSAIDs and sleep medication for 48 h prior to the fMRI visit (cf. Methods).

3.2. Behavior

HC rated slow and fast brushing as similarly pleasant (Figure 1, top panel). Within the FM patient group, slow brushing was rated as pleasant, while fast brushing was rated as unpleasant. Affective ratings to slow and fast brushing were lower in FM patients than HC. Pain was rated very low in HC, as expected (Figure 1, bottom panel). Notwithstanding, HC reported less pain to slow than to fast brushing. In FM, pain was also rated somewhat lower after slow than after fast brushing. As described in the Methods, the pain ratings were not specifically related to brush-evoked sensation but to the subjects' general pain level. In summary, the HC and FM groups differed in their ratings of touch pleasantness and ongoing pain. FM rated both slow and fast brushing as less pleasant than HC. In addition, pain ratings in FM were higher than HC.

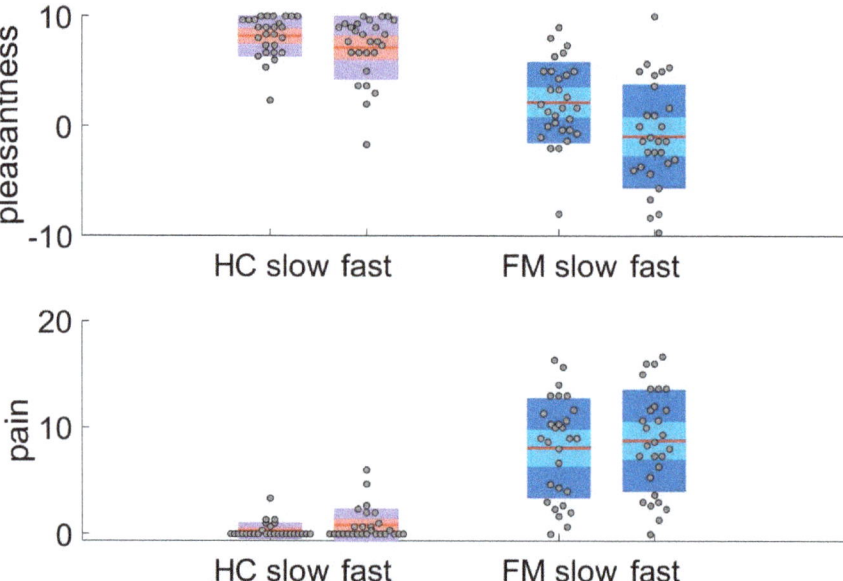

Figure 1. Ratings of touch pleasantness and pain during fMRI. Top: HC rated slow and fast brushing as similarly pleasant on a VAS (mean slow = 8.2 ± 1.9, mean fast = 7.2 ± 3, $Z = -1.6$, $p < 0.103$). FM rated slow brushing as significantly more pleasant than fast (mean slow = 2.1 ± 3.7, mean fast = −0.9 ± 4.7, $t = 4.9$, $p < 0.001$). Groups differed in their ratings of the different conditions (Mann–Whitney U test, pleasantness ratings: slow $Z = -5.7$, $p < 0.001$, fast $Z = -5.4$, $p < 0.001$). Bottom: HC rated less pain after slow than after fast brushing on a VAS (mean slow = 0.33 ± 0.04, mean fast = 0.86 ± 1.53, $Z = -2.4$, $p < 0.017$). FM rated less pain after slow than after fast brushing (mean slow = 8.3 ± 4.7, mean fast = 9 ± 4.9, $t = -2.7$, $p < 0.011$). The groups differed in their ratings of the different conditions (Mann–Whitney U test, pain ratings: slow $Z = -6.2$, $p < 0.001$, fast $Z = -5.9$, $p < 0.001$). Note that the pain ratings were not specifically related to brush-evoked sensation but to the subjects' general pain level.

3.3. Functional Imaging

Across all participants, we found a significantly stronger activation for slow compared to fast brushing in the right posterior insula (contralateral to the stimulated forearm) (Figure 2). There was no main effect of group and no difference between groups for separate slow or fast brushing.

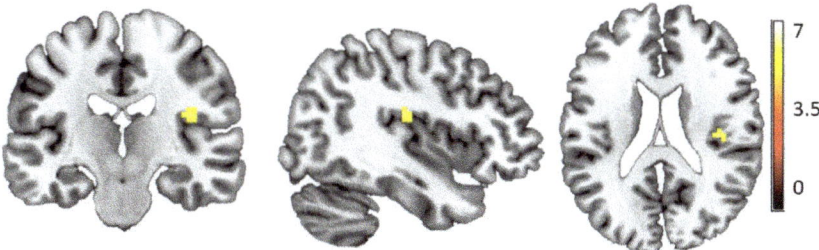

Figure 2. More activation in the posterior insula during slow brushing compared to fast brushing. In all participants, [39–1920] $t = 6.25$, $Z = 5.79$, FWE corrected at the whole-brain level $p < 0.05$, color scale depicts *t*-values for the contrast slow > fast.

Since we found a difference in ratings between HC and FM, we also explored group differences during the rating period. Activation in posterior insula was related to whether the subjects were rating on the pleasantness or the pain scale (Figure 3A). While HC showed activation in this area during pleasantness ratings and deactivation during pain ratings, patients showed the opposite pattern, i.e., deactivation during pleasantness ratings and activation during pain ratings (Figure 3B).

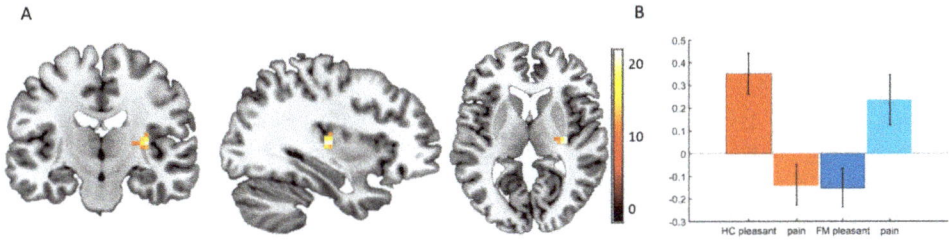

Figure 3. Insula activity differs between FM patients and HC during rating period. (**A**) Interaction group*ratings type (pleasantness and pain). During the rating period, we found a group*rating-type interaction in the posterior insula ([33–198], $F = 22.67$, $Z = 4.39$ $p = 0.001$ FWE, SVC for posterior insula), color scale depicts the F-values. (**B**) Beta values extracted from a 6 mm radius sphere around the peak of the interaction in the posterior insula [33–198].

3.4. Voxel-Based Morphometry

VBM analysis comparing HC and FM revealed reduced grey matter density in patients in the bilateral hippocampus and anterior insula. This difference was even stronger when including age as a covariate of no interest (Figure 4 and Table 2). There was no area where FM had a higher grey matter density than HC.

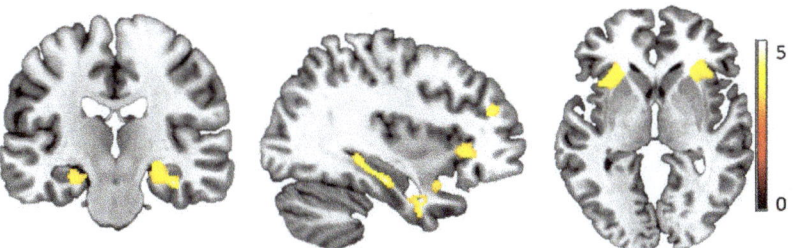

Figure 4. Reduced grey matter in FM. FM showed reduced grey matter density in bilateral insula and hippocampus ([35–19–1], $p < 0.001$, cluster size = 50), color scale depicts the *t*-values.

Table 2. Regions with reduced grey matter density in FM compared to HC. Age was included as covariate of no interest. *t*-test at the whole brain level, thresholded at $p < 0.001$ uncorrected.

Region	x	y	z	Hemi-Sphere	Cluster Size	t	p
Hippocampus	36	−22.5	−18	Right	469	4.98	>0.0001
Parahippocampal Gyrus	37.5	−31.5	−12	Right		4.68	>0.0001
	24	−19.5	−9			3.91	0.0001
	−24	−19.5	−16.5	Left	146	3.94	0.0002
Middle Frontal Gyrus	31.5	45	22.5	Right	233	4.69	>0.0001
Rectal Gyrus	3	37.5	−28.5	Right	339	4.51	>0.0001
Uncus	34.5	0	−34.5	Right	505	4.43	>0.0001
	−34.5	1.5	−28.5	Left	215	3.69	0.0003
Superior Temporal Gyrus	46.5	0	−16.5	Right		3.91	0.0001
	−40.5	6	−18	Left		3.49	0.0005
Subcallosal Gyrus	13.5	6	−19.5	Right	288	4.29	>0.0001
Anterior Cingulate	9	18	−12	Right		3.51	0.0004
Anterior Insula	−28.5	21	1.5	Left	764	4.20	>0.0001
	27	25.5	0	Right	430	4.13	0.0001
Middle Occipital Gyrus	−22.5	−88.5	4.5	Left	175	4.18	0.0001
Inferior Frontal Gyrus	37.5	24	−1.5	Right		3.77	0.0002
Cingulate Gyrus	−6	−10.5	43.5	Left	131	4.07	0.0001
	−9	−10.5	36			3.72	0.0001
Cerebellum	−22.5	−31.5	−33	Left	72	3.69	0.0003

4. Discussion

In the current study, we found intact neural processing of positive affective touch in FM patients. However, slow soft brushing was reported as less pleasant by FM patients than healthy controls. We found that FM patients differed from HC during the rating of perceived pleasantness and pain. FM patients showed deactivation in the right posterior insula during the pleasantness rating and activation during the pain rating, the opposite pattern of what was observed in the HC.

4.1. Behavior

The pathophysiology of FM is not well-understood. Both peripheral and central nervous system alterations are involved in the development and maintenance of FM. Hence, alterations in the brain including neuroinflammation and activation of glial cells, nociception-driven amplification of neural signaling (central sensitization), opioidergic dysregulation, and impaired top-down modulation were found, as well as signs of systemic low-grade inflammation (e.g., regarding cytokine profile and inflammatory lipids) and nociceptor and muscle protein changes [28–40]. In an earlier psychophysical study in FM patients, we found that pleasantness ratings to brushing were normal, but the distinction between slow CT-optimal and fast CT-suboptimal brushing was diminished [8]. In the current study, we found that while the affective touch sensitivity (slow versus fast) was preserved, the pleasantness ratings were significantly lower in FM. Despite these differences which, in part at least, could be due to the heterogeneity of the condition [41], there is likely a disturbance in the affective touch system. To confirm whether this has a peripheral involvement would require electrophysiological recordings (microneurography) from CT afferents in FM patients.

The finding that HC did not rate the pleasantness of slow and fast brushing differently needs further consideration. Although average pleasantness ratings were descriptively higher for slow than for fast brushing, they were not statistically different. Previous studies have reported that people rate slow, CT-optimal brushing velocities as more pleasant than fast, CT-non-optimal brushing [3,26,42]. However, a recent study challenged the view of an inverted U-shaped curve for pleasantness ratings that peaks at the CT-optimal velocity, suggesting that the inverted U-shape can only be found as a group average [43]. Our sample might have contained healthy individuals who did not differentiate as much between a slow and fast touch. Another, possibly complementary explanation, might be a ceiling effect. This might be driven by a number of factors; the MRI-scanner environment was loud, uncomfortable, and boring, so any positive stimulus might be evaluated as especially pleasant. In addition, the combination with a question on pain experience might drive an overly positive evaluation of the brushing stimuli.

4.2. Functional Imaging

We found differential processing during the evaluative period for the two groups and conditions. While HC showed activation in posterior insula during pleasantness evaluation and deactivation during pain evaluation, FM showed deactivation during pleasantness evaluation and activation during pain evaluation. This result should be considered preliminary as it was the result of an exploratory analysis. That the cluster of the interaction effect did not directly overlap with the main effect of slow versus fast touch was not surprising, since the evaluative processing of the current experience was a different, hierarchically higher processing, and might therefore have involved different clusters within the insula [44–48].

FM patients display hyper-sensitivity to a range of sensory stimuli [49], so it has been suggested that this might be a general hypersensitivity syndrome [50]. Our results suggest that FM patients do not exhibit hypersensitivity to pleasant touch at an early processing stage, as we found no difference in neural activation in the posterior insula. However, we found altered activation patterns during the evaluation of positive stimuli and reporting of current pain levels, suggesting dysfunctional evaluative processes. This was in line with other studies; for instance, a study in which FM patients were compared to subjects with masochistic behavior found an alteration in the late response to tactile stimulation in the primary somatosensory cortex, as measured by magnetoencephalography [51]. The amplitude of this cortical response was inversely correlated with pain catastrophizing. Dysfunctional evaluative processing of a pleasant stimulus might be associated with anhedonia in FM. FM patients are less efficient at modulating their pain perception through concomitant positive stimuli [52], however, we found a small but significant reduction in pain ratings after slow brushing (rated as pleasant by the patients). Pain catastrophizing affects pain sensitivity (i.e., pain thresholds for pressure, cold, or heat) as reported in various cohorts of patients with chronic pain [53,54]. However, correlations are moderate, and the pain sensitivity is not solely explained by psychological aspects. Moreover, catastrophizing is related to fear of pain but also these correlations are moderate [55–57].

4.3. VBM

Alterations in grey matter in many brain regions related to pain processing have been reported in several studies (for review see [58]). These include grey matter increases in the cerebellum and the striatum [59] and decreases in the brainstem, anterior and posterior cingulate cortices, prefrontal cortex, parahippocampal gyrus, and hippocampus [60,61]. For certain areas, interaction with age was also reported, e.g., increased grey matter in the insula of patients younger than 50 years [62]. In the current study, we found decreased grey matter density in FM, in the bilateral hippocampus and insula—a reduction that was more pronounced when age was included (as a covariate of no interest). However, we found no brain region where FM patients had higher grey matter density than HC.

The hippocampal grey matter is decreased in people suffering from stress [63] and post-traumatic stress disorder [64]. This is consistent with a high prevalence of early life stress and adverse events in FM [65,66]. In our FM cohort, we found high distress, pain catastrophizing and insomnia, and a low perceived state of health. The insula plays an important role in the perception of one's own body and sensations created within [48], specifically pain [67]. The anterior insula is involved in stratifying sensations into painful and non-painful [68]. The reduction in the anterior insular grey matter observed here might relate to alterations in the pain network in FM, as has been suggested previously [69].

4.4. Limitations and Future Direction

There are several limitations that need to be considered when interpreting our results. FM is a condition of highly varied symptoms and severity; therefore, patient samples tend to be heterogeneous. Larger and longitudinal studies are needed to distinguish subgroups within FM. Here, we focused on brushing for its affective attribute and link to C-tactile fibers, and questionnaires to capture the clinical characteristics, but we did not perform a detailed battery of quantitative somatosensory tests [70–72]; the combination of these could provide important insights into the peripheral nerve function, the role of top-down modulation, and the broader interplay between somatosensory and affective systems in aberrant pain states. To further disentangle perception and evaluation of sensory inputs, future studies could compare measures of hypersensitivity in the tactile domain with other sensory domains [73]. Physical activity is another important factor—while exercise leads to hypoalgesia in healthy individuals, it leads to hyperalgesia in patients with FM [74]. Further, FM patients have a heightened sensitivity to activity-related increases in pain [56]. Here, we simply asked patients to rate the extent to which pain affected their activities of daily living, leisure, and work. In future studies it would be interesting to explore this in detail using, for instance, the Sensitivity to Physical Activity (SPA) measures that are associated with clinical indices of pain hypersensitivity [75]. Another interesting future direction would be to focus on neurotransmitters such as glutamate, which is elevated in the insula in FM [11]. Glutamate could be tracked using biosensors [76] or could be measured in the brain using magnetic resonance spectroscopy [77], and these measures could then be related to behavioral and functional differences in FM patients.

Taken together, our results suggest intact early-stage sensory processing of positive tactile stimuli but dysfunctional evaluative processing. These findings contribute to our understanding of the mechanisms underlying anhedonia in FM.

Author Contributions: Conceptualization, B.G., H.O., and H.v.E.-V.; methodology, B.G., H.O., S.S.N.; software, R.B. and H.v.E.-V.; formal analysis, R.B.; investigation, S.S.N., R.B., and H.v.E.-V., B.G.; resources, B.G. and H.O.; data curation, R.B., S.S.N., H.v.E.-V., and B.G.; writing—original draft preparation, R.B.; writing—review and editing, R.B., S.S.N., H.O., and B.G.; visualization, R.B.; supervision, H.O. and B.G.; project administration, B.G.; funding acquisition, R.B., B.G., H.O., and S.S.N. All authors have read and agreed to the published version of the manuscript.

Funding: This research was funded by Research-ALF Region Östergötland awarded to H.O., S.S.N. (LIO-900631), and B.G. (LIO-700931) and the Swedish Research Council awarded to B.G. (2018-02470) and R.B. (2019-01873).

Acknowledgments: We would like to thank research nurse Eva-Britt Lind and research physiotherapist Ulrika Wentzel Olausson at the Pain and Rehabilitation Centre, University hospital, Linköping, for valuable help during the recruitment process and sample collection.

Conflicts of Interest: The authors declare no conflict of interest.

References

1. Wolfe, F.; Smythe, H.A.; Yunus, M.B.; Bennett, R.M.; Bombardier, C.; Goldenberg, D.L.; Tugwell, P.; Campbell, S.M.; Abeles, M.; Clark, P.; et al. The American College of Rheumatology 1990 Criteria for the Classification of Fibromyalgia. Report of the Multicenter Criteria Committee. *Arthritis Rheum.* **1990**, *33*, 160–172. [CrossRef] [PubMed]
2. Wolfe, F.; Ross, K.; Anderson, J.; Russell, I.J.; Hebert, L. The prevalence and characteristics of fibromyalgia in the general population. *Arthritis Rheum.* **1995**, *38*, 19–28. [CrossRef] [PubMed]
3. McGlone, F.; Wessberg, J.; Olausson, H. Discriminative and affective touch: Sensing and feeling. *Neuron* **2014**, *82*, 737–755. [CrossRef] [PubMed]
4. Löken, L.S.; Wessberg, J.; McGlone, F.; Olausson, H. Coding of pleasant touch by unmyelinated afferents in humans. *Nat. Neurosci.* **2009**, *12*, 547. [CrossRef]
5. Liljencrantz, J.; Strigo, I.; Ellingsen, D.; Krämer, H.; Lundblad, L.; Nagi, S.; Leknes, S.; Olausson, H. Slow brushing reduces heat pain in humans. *Eur. J. Pain* **2017**, *21*, 1173–1185. [CrossRef] [PubMed]
6. Nagi, S.S.; Rubin, T.K.; Chelvanayagam, D.K.; Macefield, V.G.; Mahns, D.A. Allodynia mediated by C-tactile afferents in human hairy skin. *J. Physiol.* **2011**, *589*, 4065–4075. [CrossRef]

7. Serra, J.; Collado, A.; Solà, R.; Antonelli, F.; Torres, X.; Salgueiro, M.; Quiles, C.; Bostock, H. Hyperexcitable C nociceptors in fibromyalgia. *Ann. Neurol.* **2014**, *75*, 196–208. [CrossRef]
8. Case, L.K.; Ceko, M.; Gracely, J.L.; Richards, E.A.; Olausson, H.; Bushnell, M.C. Touch Perception Altered by Chronic Pain and by Opioid Blockade. *eNeuro* **2016**, *3*, ENEURO.0138-15.2016. [CrossRef]
9. Henderson, L.A.; Gandevia, S.C.; Macefield, V.G. Somatotopic organization of the processing of muscle and cutaneous pain in the left and right insula cortex: A single-trial fMRI study. *Pain* **2007**, *128*, 20–30. [CrossRef]
10. Bjornsdotter, M.; Loken, L.; Olausson, H.; Vallbo, A.; Wessberg, J. Somatotopic organization of gentle touch processing in the posterior insular cortex. *J. Neurosci.* **2009**, *29*, 9314–9320. [CrossRef]
11. Harris, R.E.; Sundgren, P.C.; Pang, Y.; Hsu, M.; Petrou, M.; Kim, S.H.; McLean, S.A.; Gracely, R.H.; Clauw, D.J. Dynamic levels of glutamate within the insula are associated with improvements in multiple pain domains in fibromyalgia. *Arthritis Rheum.* **2008**, *58*, 903–907. [CrossRef] [PubMed]
12. Wolfe, F.; Clauw, D.J.; Fitzcharles, M.A.; Goldenberg, D.L.; Hauser, W.; Katz, R.L.; Mease, P.J.; Russell, A.S.; Russell, I.J.; Walitt, B. 2016 Revisions to the 2010/2011 fibromyalgia diagnostic criteria. *Semin. Arthritis Rheum.* **2016**, *46*, 319–329. [CrossRef] [PubMed]
13. Arnold, L.M.; Bennett, R.M.; Crofford, L.J.; Dean, L.E.; Clauw, D.J.; Goldenberg, D.L.; Fitzcharles, M.A.; Paiva, E.S.; Staud, R.; Sarzi-Puttini, P.; et al. AAPT Diagnostic Criteria for Fibromyalgia. *J. Pain* **2019**, *20*, 611–628. [CrossRef]
14. Lisspers, J.; Nygren, A.; Söderman, E. Hospital Anxiety and Depression Scale (HAD): Some psychometric data for a Swedish sample. *Acta Psychiatr. Scand.* **1997**, *96*, 281–286. [CrossRef] [PubMed]
15. Zigmond, A.S.; Snaith, R.P. The hospital anxiety and depression scale. *Acta Psychiatr. Scand.* **1983**, *67*, 361–370. [CrossRef] [PubMed]
16. Bjelland, I.; Dahl, A.A.; Haug, T.T.; Neckelmann, D. The validity of the Hospital Anxiety and Depression Scale. An updated literature review. *J. Psychosom. Res.* **2002**, *52*, 69–77. [CrossRef]
17. Bastien, C.H.; Vallieres, A.; Morin, C.M. Validation of the Insomnia Severity Index as an outcome measure for insomnia research. *Sleep Med.* **2001**, *2*, 297–307. [CrossRef]
18. Morin, C.M.; Belleville, G.; Belanger, L.; Ivers, H. The Insomnia Severity Index: Psychometric indicators to detect insomnia cases and evaluate treatment response. *Sleep* **2011**, *34*, 601–608. [CrossRef]
19. Miro, J.; Nieto, R.; Huguet, A. The Catalan version of the Pain Catastrophizing Scale: A useful instrument to assess catastrophic thinking in whiplash patients. *J. Pain* **2008**, *9*, 397–406. [CrossRef]
20. Sullivan, M.; Bishop, S.; Pivik, J. The Pain catastrophizing scale: Development and validation. *Psychol. Assess.* **1995**, *7*, 524–532. [CrossRef]
21. Kemani, M.K.; Grimby-Ekman, A.; Lundgren, J.; Sullivan, M.; Lundberg, M. Factor structure and internal consistency of a Swedish version of the Pain Catastrophizing Scale. *Acta Anaesthesiol. Scand.* **2019**, *63*, 259–266. [CrossRef] [PubMed]
22. EuroQol. EuroQol: A new facility for the measurement of health-related quality of life. *Health Policy* **1990**, *16*, 199–208. [CrossRef]
23. Brooks, R. EuroQol: The current state of play. *Health Policy* **1996**, *37*, 53–72. [CrossRef]
24. Dolan, P.; Sutton, M. Mapping visual analogue scale health state valuations onto standard gamble and time trade-off values. *Soc. Sci. Med.* **1997**, *44*, 1519–1530. [CrossRef]
25. Ashburner, J.; Friston, K.J. Unified segmentation. *Neuroimage* **2005**, *26*, 839–851. [CrossRef]
26. Morrison, I.; Bjornsdotter, M.; Olausson, H. Vicarious responses to social touch in posterior insular cortex are tuned to pleasant caressing speeds. *J. Neurosci.* **2011**, *31*, 9554–9562. [CrossRef]
27. Larsson, M.B.; Tillisch, K.; Craig, A.; Engström, M.; Labus, J.; Naliboff, B.; Lundberg, P.; Ström, M.; Mayer, E.A.; Walter, S.A. Brain responses to visceral stimuli reflect visceral sensitivity thresholds in patients with irritable bowel syndrome. *Gastroenterology* **2012**, *142*, 463–472.e3. [CrossRef]
28. Backryd, E.; Tanum, L.; Lind, A.L.; Larsson, A.; Gordh, T. Evidence of both systemic inflammation and neuroinflammation in fibromyalgia patients, as assessed by a multiplex protein panel applied to the cerebrospinal fluid and to plasma. *J. Pain Res.* **2017**, *10*, 515–525. [CrossRef]
29. Furer, V.; Hazan, E.; Mor, A.; Segal, M.; Katav, A.; Aloush, V.; Elkayam, O.; George, J.; Ablin, J.N. Elevated Levels of Eotaxin-2 in Serum of Fibromyalgia Patients. *Pain Res. Manag.* **2018**, *2018*, 7257681. [CrossRef]
30. Rodriguez-Pinto, I.; Agmon-Levin, N.; Howard, A.; Shoenfeld, Y. Fibromyalgia and cytokines. *Immunol. Lett.* **2014**, *161*, 200–203. [CrossRef]

31. Stensson, N.; Ghafouri, N.; Ernberg, M.; Mannerkorpi, K.; Kosek, E.; Gerdle, B.; Ghafouri, B. The Relationship of Endocannabinoidome Lipid Mediators With Pain and Psychological Stress in Women With Fibromyalgia: A Case-Control Study. *J. Pain* **2018**, *19*, 1318–1328. [CrossRef] [PubMed]
32. Sluka, K.A.; Clauw, D.J. Neurobiology of fibromyalgia and chronic widespread pain. *Neuroscience* **2016**, *338*, 114–129. [CrossRef] [PubMed]
33. Schrepf, A.; Harper, D.E.; Harte, S.E.; Wang, H.; Ichesco, E.; Hampson, J.P.; Zubieta, J.K.; Clauw, D.J.; Harris, R.E. Endogenous opioidergic dysregulation of pain in fibromyalgia: A PET and fMRI study. *Pain* **2016**, *157*, 2217–2225. [CrossRef] [PubMed]
34. Üçeyler, N.; Sommer, C. Small nerve fiber pathology. In *Fibromylagia Syndrome and Widespread Pain—From Construction to Relevant Recognition*; Häuser, W., Perrot, S., Eds.; Wolters Kluwer: Philadelphia, PA, USA, 2018; pp. 204–214.
35. Gerdle, B.; Larsson, B. Muscle. In *Fibromyalgia Syndrome and Widespread Pain—From Construction to Relevant Recognition*; Häuser, W., Perrot, S., Eds.; Wolters Kluwer: Philadelphia, PA, USA, 2018; pp. 215–231.
36. Albrecht, D.S.; Forsberg, A.; Sandstrom, A.; Bergan, C.; Kadetoff, D.; Protsenko, E.; Lampa, J.; Lee, Y.C.; Hoglund, C.O.; Catana, C.; et al. Brain glial activation in fibromyalgia—A multi-site positron emission tomography investigation. *Brain Behav. Immun.* **2019**, *75*, 72–83. [CrossRef]
37. Jensen, K.B.; Kosek, E.; Petzke, F.; Carville, S.; Fransson, P.; Marcus, H.; Williams, S.C.R.; Choy, E.; Giesecke, T.; Mainguy, Y.; et al. Evidence of dysfunctional pain inhibition in Fibromyalgia reflected in rACC during provoked pain. *Pain* **2009**, *144*, 95–100. [CrossRef]
38. Olausson, P.; Gerdle, B.; Ghafouri, N.; Larsson, B.; Ghafouri, B. Identification of proteins from interstitium of trapezius muscle in women with chronic myalgia using microdialysis in combination with proteomics. *PLoS ONE* **2012**, *7*, e52560. [CrossRef]
39. Olausson, P.; Gerdle, B.; Ghafouri, N.; Sjostrom, D.; Blixt, E.; Ghafouri, B. Protein alterations in women with chronic widespread pain—An explorative proteomic study of the trapezius muscle. *Sci. Rep.* **2015**, *5*, 11894. [CrossRef]
40. Hadrevi, J.; Ghafouri, B.; Larsson, B.; Gerdle, B.; Hellstrom, F. Multivariate modeling of proteins related to trapezius myalgia, a comparative study of female cleaners with or without pain. *PLoS ONE* **2013**, *8*, e73285. [CrossRef]
41. Hurtig, I.M.; Raak, R.I.; Kendall, S.A.; Gerdle, B.; Wahren, L.K. Quantitative sensory testing in fibromyalgia patients and in healthy subjects: Identification of subgroups. *Clin. J. Pain* **2001**, *17*, 316–322. [CrossRef]
42. Olausson, H.; Wessberg, J.; Morrison, I.; McGlone, F.; Vallbo, A. The neurophysiology of unmyelinated tactile afferents. *Neurosci. Biobehav. Rev.* **2010**, *34*, 185–191. [CrossRef]
43. Croy, I.; Bierling, A.; Sailer, U.; Ackerley, R. Individual variability of pleasantness ratings to stroking touch over different velocities. *Neuroscience* **2020**, in press. [CrossRef] [PubMed]
44. Frot, M.; Faillenot, I.; Mauguière, F. Processing of nociceptive input from posterior to anterior insula in humans. *Hum. Brain Mapp.* **2014**, *35*, 5486–5499. [CrossRef] [PubMed]
45. Kurth, F.; Zilles, K.; Fox, P.T.; Laird, A.R.; Eickhoff, S.B. A link between the systems: Functional differentiation and integration within the human insula revealed by meta-analysis. *Brain Struct. Funct.* **2010**, *214*, 519–534. [CrossRef] [PubMed]
46. Uddin, L.Q.; Kinnison, J.; Pessoa, L.; Anderson, M.L. Beyond the tripartite cognition–emotion–interoception model of the human insular cortex. *J. Cognit. Neurosci.* **2014**, *26*, 16–27. [CrossRef]
47. Evrard, H.C. The organization of the primate insular cortex. *Front. Neuroanat.* **2019**, *13*, 43. [CrossRef]
48. Craig, A.D. How do you feel—Now? The anterior insula and human awareness. *Nat. Rev. Neurosci.* **2009**, *10*, 59–70. [CrossRef]
49. Geisser, M.E.; Glass, J.M.; Rajcevska, L.D.; Clauw, D.J.; Williams, D.A.; Kileny, P.R.; Gracely, R.H. A psychophysical study of auditory and pressure sensitivity in patients with fibromyalgia and healthy controls. *J. Pain* **2008**, *9*, 417–422. [CrossRef]
50. B Yunus, M. Editorial review (thematic issue: An update on central sensitivity syndromes and the issues of nosology and psychobiology). *Curr. Rheumatol. Rev.* **2015**, *11*, 70–85. [CrossRef]
51. Pollok, B.; Krause, V.; Legrain, V.; Ploner, M.; Freynhagen, R.; Melchior, I.; Schnitzler, A. Differential effects of painful and non-painful stimulation on tactile processing in fibromyalgia syndrome and subjects with masochistic behaviour. *PLoS ONE* **2010**, *5*, e15804. [CrossRef]

52. Kamping, S.; Bomba, I.C.; Kanske, P.; Diesch, E.; Flor, H. Deficient modulation of pain by a positive emotional context in fibromyalgia patients. *PAIN®* **2013**, *154*, 1846–1855. [CrossRef]
53. Wallin, M.; Liedberg, G.; Börsbo, B.; Gerdle, B. Thermal detection and pain thresholds but not pressure pain thresholds are correlated with psychological factors in women with chronic whiplash-associated pain. *Clin. J. Pain* **2012**, *28*, 211–221. [CrossRef] [PubMed]
54. Grundström, H.; Larsson, B.; Arendt-Nielsen, L.; Gerdle, B.; Kjølhede, P. Pain catastrophizing is associated with pain thresholds for heat, cold and pressure in women with chronic pelvic pain. *Scand. J. Pain* **2020**, in press.
55. Martínez, M.P.; Sánchez, A.I.; Miró, E.; Medina, A.; Lami, M.J. The relationship between the fear-avoidance model of pain and personality traits in fibromyalgia patients. *J. Clin. Psychol. Med. Settings* **2011**, *18*, 380–391. [CrossRef]
56. Lambin, D.I.; Thibault, P.; Simmonds, M.; Lariviere, C.; Sullivan, M.J. Repetition-induced activity-related summation of pain in patients with fibromyalgia. *Pain* **2011**, *152*, 1424–1430. [CrossRef]
57. Burri, A.; Ogata, S.; Rice, D.; Williams, F. Pain catastrophizing, neuroticism, fear of pain, and anxiety: Defining the genetic and environmental factors in a sample of female twins. *PLoS ONE* **2018**, *13*, e0194562. [CrossRef]
58. Shi, H.; Yuan, C.; Dai, Z.; Ma, H.; Sheng, L. Gray matter abnormalities associated with fibromyalgia: A meta-analysis of voxel-based morphometric studies. *Semin. Arthritis Rheum.* **2016**, *46*, 330–337. [CrossRef]
59. Schmidt-Wilcke, T.; Luerding, R.; Weigand, T.; Jürgens, T.; Schuierer, G.; Leinisch, E.; Bogdahn, U. Striatal grey matter increase in patients suffering from fibromyalgia—A voxel-based morphometry study. *Pain* **2007**, *132*, S109–S116. [CrossRef]
60. Burgmer, M.; Gaubitz, M.; Konrad, C.; Wrenger, M.; Hilgart, S.; Heuft, G.; Pfleiderer, B. Decreased gray matter volumes in the cingulo-frontal cortex and the amygdala in patients with fibromyalgia. *Psychosom. Med.* **2009**, *71*, 566–573. [CrossRef]
61. Fallon, N.; Alghamdi, J.; Chiu, Y.; Sluming, V.; Nurmikko, T.; Stancak, A. Structural alterations in brainstem of fibromyalgia syndrome patients correlate with sensitivity to mechanical pressure. *NeuroImage Clin.* **2013**, *3*, 163–170. [CrossRef]
62. Ceko, M.; Bushnell, M.C.; Fitzcharles, M.-A.; Schweinhardt, P. Fibromyalgia interacts with age to change the brain. *NeuroImage Clin.* **2013**, *3*, 249–260. [CrossRef]
63. Gianaros, P.J.; Jennings, J.R.; Sheu, L.K.; Greer, P.J.; Kuller, L.H.; Matthews, K.A. Prospective reports of chronic life stress predict decreased grey matter volume in the hippocampus. *Neuroimage* **2007**, *35*, 795–803. [CrossRef]
64. Felmingham, K.; Williams, L.M.; Whitford, T.J.; Falconer, E.; Kemp, A.H.; Peduto, A.; Bryant, R.A. Duration of posttraumatic stress disorder predicts hippocampal grey matter loss. *Neuroreport* **2009**, *20*, 1402–1406. [CrossRef]
65. Haviland, M.G.; Morton, K.R.; Oda, K.; Fraser, G.E. Traumatic experiences, major life stressors, and self-reporting a physician-given fibromyalgia diagnosis. *Psychiatry Res.* **2010**, *177*, 335–341. [CrossRef]
66. Anderberg, U.; Marteinsdottir, I.; Theorell, T.; Von Knorring, L. The impact of life events in female patients with fibromyalgia and in female healthy controls. *Eur. Psychiatry* **2000**, *15*, 295–301. [CrossRef]
67. Segerdahl, A.R.; Mezue, M.; Okell, T.W.; Farrar, J.T.; Tracey, I. The dorsal posterior insula subserves a fundamental role in human pain. *Nat. Neurosci.* **2015**, *18*, 499–500. [CrossRef]
68. Wiech, K.; Lin, C.-s.; Brodersen, K.H.; Bingel, U.; Ploner, M.; Tracey, I. Anterior insula integrates information about salience into perceptual decisions about pain. *J. Neurosci.* **2010**, *30*, 16324–16331. [CrossRef]
69. Cagnie, B.; Coppieters, I.; Denecker, S.; Six, J.; Danneels, L.; Meeus, M. Central sensitization in fibromyalgia? A systematic review on structural and functional brain MRI. *Semin. Arthritis Rheum.* **2014**, *44*, 68–75. [CrossRef]
70. Uddin, Z.; MacDermid, J.C.; Ham, H.H. Test–retest reliability and validity of normative cut-offs of the two devices measuring touch threshold: Weinstein Enhanced Sensory Test and Pressure-Specified Sensory Device. *Hand Ther.* **2014**, *19*, 3–10. [CrossRef]
71. Rolke, R.; Baron, R.; Maier, C.A.; Tölle, T.; Treede, R.-D.; Beyer, A.; Binder, A.; Birbaumer, N.; Birklein, F.; Bötefür, I. Quantitative sensory testing in the German Research Network on Neuropathic Pain (DFNS): Standardized protocol and reference values. *Pain* **2006**, *123*, 231–243. [CrossRef]

72. Pickering, G.; Achard, A.; Corriger, A.; Sickout-Arondo, S.; Macian, N.; Leray, V.; Lucchini, C.; Cardot, J.M.; Pereira, B. Electrochemical Skin Conductance and Quantitative Sensory Testing on Fibromyalgia. *Pain Pract.* **2020**, *20*, 348–356. [CrossRef]
73. Wilbarger, J.L.; Cook, D.B. Multisensory hypersensitivity in women with fibromyalgia: Implications for well being and intervention. *Arch. Phys. Med. Rehabilit.* **2011**, *92*, 653–656. [CrossRef]
74. Vierck, C.J., Jr.; Staud, R.; Price, D.D.; Cannon, R.L.; Mauderli, A.P.; Martin, A.D. The effect of maximal exercise on temporal summation of second pain (windup) in patients with fibromyalgia syndrome. *J. Pain* **2001**, *2*, 334–344. [CrossRef]
75. Woznowski-Vu, A.; Uddin, Z.; Flegg, D.; Aternali, A.; Wickens, R.; Sullivan, M.J.; Sweet, S.N.; Skou, S.T.; Wideman, T.H. Comparing Novel and Existing Measures of Sensitivity to Physical Activity Among People With Chronic Musculoskeletal Pain. *Clin. J. Pain* **2019**, *35*, 656–667. [CrossRef]
76. Schultz, J.; Uddin, Z.; Singh, G.; Howlader, M.M. Glutamate sensing in biofluids: Recent advances and research challenges of electrochemical sensors. *Analyst* **2020**, *145*, 321–347. [CrossRef]
77. Gleich, T.; Deserno, L.; Lorenz, R.C.; Boehme, R.; Pankow, A.; Buchert, R.; Kühn, S.; Heinz, A.; Schlagenhauf, F.; Gallinat, J. Prefrontal and striatal glutamate differently relate to striatal dopamine: Potential regulatory mechanisms of striatal presynaptic dopamine function? *J. Neurosci.* **2015**, *35*, 9615–9621. [CrossRef]

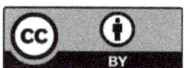

© 2020 by the authors. Licensee MDPI, Basel, Switzerland. This article is an open access article distributed under the terms and conditions of the Creative Commons Attribution (CC BY) license (http://creativecommons.org/licenses/by/4.0/).

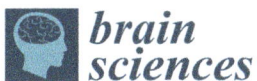

Article

Effect of Psycho-Regulatory Massage Therapy on Pain and Depression in Women with Chronic and/or Somatoform Back Pain: A Randomized Controlled Trial

Sabine B.-E. Baumgart [1,*], Anja Baumbach-Kraft [2] and Juergen Lorenz [3]

[1] Faculty of Medicine, Institute for Health and Nursing Sciences, Martin Luther University Halle-Wittenberg, 06108 Halle, Germany
[2] M.Sc. Public Health, 24105 Kiel, Germany; baumbach.anja@gmail.com
[3] Department of Biomedical Engineering, Faculty of Life Science, University of Applied Sciences, 21033 Hamburg, Germany; juergen.lorenz@haw-hamburg.de
* Correspondence: edelbaumgart@web.de

Received: 9 September 2020; Accepted: 30 September 2020; Published: 12 October 2020

Abstract: Chronic unspecific back pain (cBP) is often associated with depressive symptoms, negative body perception, and abnormal interoception. Given the general failure of surgery in cBP, treatment guidelines focus on conservative therapies. Neurophysiological evidence indicates that C-tactile fibers associated with the oxytonergic system can be activated by slow superficial stroking of the skin in the back, shoulder, neck, and dorsal limb areas. We hypothesize that, through recruitment of C-tactile fibers, psycho-regulatory massage therapy (PRMT) can reduce pain in patients with cBP. In our study, 66 patients were randomized to PRMT or CMT (classical massage therapy) over a 12-week period and tested by questionnaires regarding pain (HSAL= Hamburger Schmerz Adjektiv Liste; Hamburg Pain adjective list), depression (BDI-II = Beck depression inventory), and disability (ODI = Oswestry Disability Index). In all outcome measures, patients receiving PRMT improved significantly more than did those receiving CMT. The mean values of the HSAL sensory subscale decreased by −51.5% in the PRMT group compared to −6.7% in the CMT group. Depressive symptoms were reduced by −55.69% (PRMT) and −3.1% (CMT), respectively. The results suggest that the superiority of PRMT over CMT may rely on its ability to activate the C-tactile fibers of superficial skin layers, recruiting the oxytonergic system.

Keywords: massage therapy; chronic back pain; depression; oxytocin; C-tactile fibers; somatoform pain (ICD 10); somatic symptom disorder (DSM-5)

1. Introduction

Chronic back pain (cBP) has a leading position worldwide in disease-related disability and loss of quality of life [1]. It represents a common health problem, especially among women. According to a GEDA ("Gesundheit in Deutschland Aktuell", current state of health in Germany) survey from 2009/2010, one in four women reported suffering cBP (lasting >3 months) within the last 12 months [2]. Modern recommendations by national and international health organizations focus on non-drug therapy options in the treatment of chronic (non-specific) back pain. A variety of treatment modalities are suggested, including physical and rehabilitation interventions [3] and instrument-based techniques such as transcutaneous electrical nerve stimulation (TENS) [4], acupuncture [5], low-level laser therapy (LLLT) [6], and shock wave therapy [7]. Additional treatment with pain-relieving medication is recommended. Surgery is not recommended because there is little evidence of its effectiveness [5,8,9]. Chou et al. [10] underlined these recommendations and showed that psychological impairments, e.g., sleep disorders, mood fluctuation, depression, and listlessness, are frequent co-morbidities of chronic pain. A central characteristic of patients with chronic pain is their negative body perception [11], inhibiting cognitive access to therapy [12–14].

In the 1980s, Groddek and Dogs integrated massage therapy as a form of body therapy into the treatment of chronic pain to gain direct access to the patient's emotions via their skin and its nervous system, thus facilitating positive body perception and cognitive-behavioral treatment [15,16]. Berg et al. and Listing et al. [17,18] showed how professional therapeutic touch in the form of massage can reduce the physical and psychological symptoms of patients with pain and/or depression. A reduction in pain, mood disorders, and listlessness and fatigue was reported. Furthermore, general psychological tension was reduced, and well-being was increased. Baumgart et al. reviewed randomized controlled trials (RCTs) published from 1996 to 2009 that investigated the effectiveness of massage for patients with depression both as the main diagnosis and a co-morbidity [16]. The authors concluded that the effectiveness of massage therapy depends on the design of the parameters of (a) pressure, (b) speed, (c) direction, and (d) rhythm [14,18–22]. Studies on the effects of oxytocin and its interactions with the neuro-physiological system have provided possible explanations for the effect of touch or massage therapy in chronic pain (with and without depression) [23]. In their study, Walker and McGlone illustrated the connection between the type of touch (effect parameters: pressure and time), its neurological transmission of stimuli via C-tactile fibers, and the significance of oxytocin with regard to pain-relieving effects [24]. C-tactile afferent fibers mediate pleasantness of touch and serve a fundamental role in the hedonic function of tactile sensation [25]. Kane and Terrel emphasized the role of touch for child development and propagated the integration of touch into the treatment of developmental trauma [26]. Experimental evidence indicates that activation of C-tactile fibers can significantly alleviate muscle pain [27]. The stimulus of a gentle or moderate touch, transduced in the skin by C-tactile fibers, is transmitted via ascending spinothalamic pathways to the insular cortex, an area of the limbic system. Through connections with the paraventricular nucleus, the thalamus stimulates the synthesis of oxytocin when a touch is perceived as pleasant [23,28,29].

Based on these considerations, we hypothesize that pain experience and depressive symptoms can be reduced and physical capacity can be improved by gentle massage that is optimized to activate C-tactile skin afferents. The aim of this study is to examine the effect of both classical and psycho-regulatory massage in patients with cBP on pain experience, depressive symptoms, and physical capacity.

2. Materials and Methods

The study was conducted as a double-blind RCT. The study is registered in the German Registry for Clinical Studies (DRKS00006876), and the protocol was approved by the ethics committee of the University of Halle (Saale), Germany (Nr. 2014-22).

2.1. Eligibility Criteria

The eligibility criteria and baseline data were assessed prior to randomization. The inclusion and exclusion criteria can be found in Table 1 and were defined via extensive literature research. The diagnosis M54 in the ICD-10 (International Statistical Classification of Diseases and Related Health Problems) represents a composite of diagnoses related to back pain.

Table 1. List of eligibility criteria for study participation.

Inclusion Criteria	Exclusion Criteria
• Back pain diagnosis according to the ICD-10 code: M54 and F45, medically certified • Pain duration of >6 months • Patient age 18–75 years • Voluntary participation in the study • Sufficient knowledge of German to understand the questionnaires	• Limited ability for consent to study participation • Inflammatory disorders • Open wounds • Ongoing application for pension

Clear diagnosis of chronic pain is difficult, since 90% of the diagnoses do not reveal any apparent clinical findings [30,31]; thus, chronic pain is primarily defined by the duration of the pain [32,33]. Since chronic pain can lead to psychological co-morbidity [34], the diagnostic group of somatoform disorders (ICD-10, F45) was also included. These disorders are generally defined by the occurrence of physical problems without a clear somatic diagnosis.

2.2. Participants

We conducted 107 recruitment interviews. Of these, 41 patients did not participate for the following reasons: $n = 16$ did not meet eligibility criteria, $n = 3$ stated that the number of interventions was too high, $n = 11$ were not comfortable with the nudity required for massage therapy, $n = 8$ found that the questionnaires were too complicated, and $n = 3$ did not want to use massage oil. Overall, $n = 66$ patients were randomized into either the intervention or control group using hidden lots covered in envelopes. One patient was excluded prior to the first treatment due to acute illness; 61 patients completed the treatment. Two patients in each treatment group discontinued the treatments without giving any reason (see Figure 1).

2.3. Interventions

Interventions took place in the physiotherapy practice operated by the principle investigator (SB). The outpatient setting was chosen to maximize external validity. The intervention group received psycho-regulatory massage therapy (PRMT) and the control group received classical massage therapy (CMT). Patients were blinded towards the type of massage they received. However, they were aware of the study's aim to compare the two types of massage. Data analysis was blind towards a patient's treatment method. All therapists employed in the practice participated in the study ($n = 7$). The design of effect parameters differed between the intervention and control groups in terms of pressure, speed, direction, and rhythm [12,14], as shown in Table 2. The interventions also differed in respect to the target organ and body areas treated. PRMT targets the skin and the superficial fascia, whereas CMT targets all layers of the tissue, including the periosteum. The PRMT unfolds from three partial massages to a full body massage. It is applied with warm oil in both supine and prone body positions and involves soft to moderate intensities of continuous slow strokes. They are uninterrupted throughout the entire session except during the change from supine to prone body position. The therapist does not touch the different body parts in separate sequences, but moves in harmonious transitions from limbs to trunk to create a whole-body experience. An extended description of the PRMT technique is added as supplemental material. In contrast, CMT is applied to the back alone and extends from the sacrum to the neck.

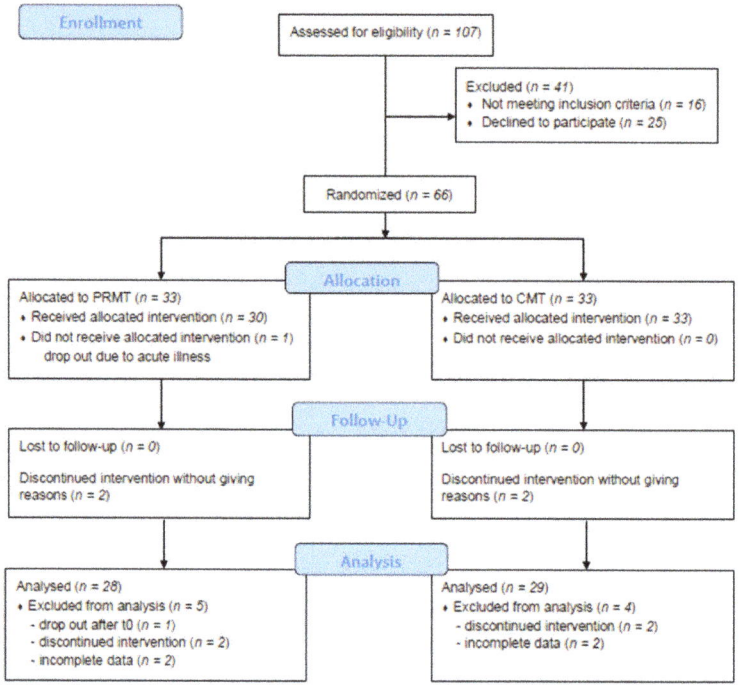

Figure 1. CONSORT (Consolidated Standards of Reporting Trials) flow chart of participants in this study comparing PRMT (psycho-regulatory massage therapy) and CMT (classical massage therapy).

Table 2. Effect parameters of the interventions.

Parameters	PRMT	CMT
Pressure	• soft to moderate	• soft to strong
Speed	• continuously decreasing to a speed of 10–3 cm per second	• a slow speed is recommended for pain reduction • not clearly defined, depends on training and individual therapist
Direction	• Body areas are connected • ending with cranial to caudal strokes	• depends on therapist's training • from the origin to the beginning of a muscle
Rhythm	• harmonious and constant contact with the patients until the end of the treatment	• not defined

PRMT, psyochregulatory massage therapy; CMT, classical massage therapy.

The intervention group was treated by seven therapists who received professional training to standardize the performance of PRMT, which was applied for 30 to 60 min [35,36]. The control group received 20 min of CMT, which was not standardized but applied individually, reflecting standard care within the German statutory health insurance scheme. All treatments were applied non-verbally in a closed therapy room with only the patient and therapist present. Patients were treated by the same therapist during the whole study period, for optimal therapeutic effectiveness [18,21]. Each group received 10 treatments overall, which were scheduled twice a week.

2.4. Data collection

After 3 months, follow-up data were collected. Figure 2 shows the structure and course of the study. Data were collected via questionnaires, handed out by the therapists and filled by the patients themselves. Baseline data (T0) were collected prior to randomization and the first intervention. At T1 (5th treatment), T2 (10th treatment), and at follow-up (T3), data were collected after the interventions.

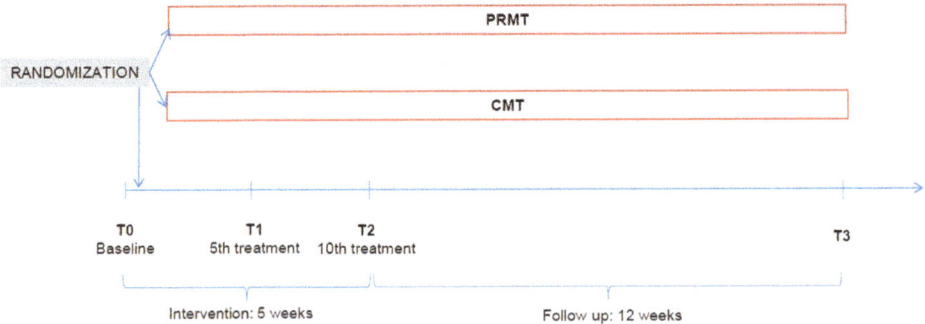

Figure 2. Study timeline (T, time of measurement; PRMT, psychoregulatory massage therapy; CMT, classical massage therapy).

Pain was assessed using the Hamburg Pain Adjective List (Hamburger Schmerz Adjektiv Liste, HSAL), a multi-dimensional questionnaire for pain experience in adults with acute or chronic pain. The HSAL consists of 37 adjectives, 21 of those describing the affective experience of pain (pain suffering + pain anxiety) and 16 describing the sensory experience of pain (pain rhythm + pain acuity). Each item can be answered on a scale from 0 (not correct at all) to 6 (completely correct), and the answers are added up to create a total score (maximum of 222, corresponding to a maximum of pain) [37]. The validity of the HSAL has been assessed by several studies in different clinical situations (Cronbach's alpha of the primary scales is between 0.80 and 0.90) [38]. The HSAL questionnaire is especially suitable in connection with psychiatric scales (depression, anxiety) and also has good applicability for monitoring patient health.

Depressiveness was measured using the Beck Depression Inventory (BDI-II), scaling 0–3 for each item; the maximum overall score is 63 points [39,40]. The severity of depression is categorized into five groups:

0–8   no depression;
9–13   minimal depression;
14–19   mild depression;
20–28   moderate depression;
29–63   severe depression [41].

The clinical relevance of the respective changes in depression was assessed according to the criteria of Hiroe et al. [42]. Accordingly, a 5-point change in BDI-II score indicates minimal relevance, 10–19 points is moderate, and more than 20 points corresponds to a strong effect.

Quality of life was measured using the Oswestry Disability Index (ODI), a self-rating questionnaire about disability in patients with back pain [43]. The questionnaire consists of 10 items, which are categorized into (1) physical complaints (or disability), (2) activity, and (3) participation according to the International Classification of Functioning, Disability and Health (ICF). A maximum score of 50 indicates maximum impairment. The scores are then converted into percentages depending on the number of questions answered. Mannion et al. [44,45] and Hooff et al. [46] investigated the validity of the German version. Their results showed that the ODI is a good measurement tool for assessing a patient's disability due to back pain (Cronbach's alpha = 0.90). The total ODI score represents a percentage and is interpreted as follows:

0–2 minimal disability (all activities of daily living (ADL) are mostly possible, often no therapy necessary, activation of life is enough);

21–40 moderate disability (participation is already limited and incapacity to work often occurs, conservative treatment);

41–60 severe disability (pain is the main problem and ADL are affected, intensive diagnostics are necessary);

61–80 crippled (all areas of life are affected);

81–100 bedridden or the patient exaggerates [47,48].

2.5. Sample Size and Randomization

For sample size calculation on the basis of overall pain experience as the primary outcome, alpha was set to 5%, statistical power should be at least 90% (SD 2.0), and the drop-out rate was expected to be 20%, resulting in a group size of $n = 33$. Block randomization was carried out with a block size of 10 by an independent statistician from University of Halle, Saale (Germany).

2.6. Statistical Analysis

Given the ordinal data type of all questionnaires (HSAL-total, HSAL-affective, HSAL-sensory, BDI-II-score, and ODI (%)) that were, in at least one session, not normally distributed, as tested with the Kolmogorov–Smirnov test, we applied the Wilcoxon rank-sum test for two independent samples to analyze group differences (CMT vs. PRMT) at baseline (T0) and to test the magnitude of change from baseline to the T1, T2, and T3 time points (SPSS, Version 26). A significant difference (two-tailed test) was accepted at p-values below 0.05. To test the effect of sessions, we applied the Friedmann ANOVA test separately for CMT and PRMT. In case of significance, we used the Wilcoxon test for paired samples. According to the total of six comparisons, we used Bonferroni correction, resulting in a p-value of 0.008 as the threshold for significance.

3. Results

The results of the non-parametric comparison using the Wilcoxon rank-sum test for two independent samples are summarized in Table 3 for all study parameters. The baseline condition (T0) yielded non-significant differences for all questionnaire scores.

HSAL total, affective, and sensory scores for pain: The total scores and the affective and sensory subscores of HSAL were significantly smaller in the T2 and T3 sessions in the PRMT group compared to the CMT group. No difference appeared in session T1. The Friedmann ANOVA yielded a non-significant effect of treatment session for CMT in HSAL-Total ($p = 0.56$), weak significance for HSAL-Affective that failed to reach the significance criterion in any of the six comparisons, and an absence of significance for HSAL-Sensory ($p = 0.127$). In contrast, all HSAL parameters were statistically significant for the effect of treatment session in PRMT ($p < 0.001$). Post hoc Wilcoxon testing revealed significant decreases in all HSAL parameters for comparisons T3 vs. T0, T4 vs. T0, T3 vs. T2, and T4 vs. T2 ($p < 0.001$; Bonferroni-corrected).

BDI-II score for depression: PRMT reduced the intensity of depression more than CMT already during T1, but more strongly during sessions T2 and T3. The Friedman ANOVA resulted in a significant session effect in CMT ($p = 0.03$); however, no post hoc comparison reached the Bonferroni-corrected threshold criterion. In contrast, PRMT had a significant effect of session with statistically significant post hoc Wilcoxon testing in all six comparisons ($p < 0.001$): T0 vs. T1, T0 vs. T2, T0 vs. T3, T1 vs. T2, T1 vs. T3, and T2 vs. T3. Thus, the BDI-II score continuously decreased over the three months of treatment. Overall, the severity of depression decreased by 55.69% with PRMT, from a moderate to minimal level of severity on average [45]. Under CMT, the mean BDI-II score changed by −3.1% over the whole study period.

Table 3. Results (mean and SD) for pain experience (HSAL total score and affective and sensory subscales), depressive symptoms (BDI-II), and disability (ODI); results of the Wilcoxon rank-sum test for independent samples tested for effect of treatment (PRMT vs. CMT) and p-values for two-tailed comparisons.

		T0	T1	T2	T3
	CMT	108.72	113.34	104.76	102.62
	SD	51.86	61.75	62	61.92
	PRMT	124.82	115.04	72.14	67.32
	SD	57.81	51.38	36.16	32.86
HSAL-Total	Wilcoxon_Z	−1.76	−1.04	−4.47	−3.65
	p	n.s.	n.s.	<0.001	<0.001
	CMT	66.38	67.03	61.79	60.86
	SD	34.79	38.7	38.28	38.49
	PRMT	75.86	70.39	44.75	43.93
	SD	33.13	30.68	23.3	21.83
HSAL-Affective	Wilcoxon Z	−0.84	−1.763	−3.54	−3.38
	p	n.s.	n.s.	<0.001	<0.001
	CMT	44.66	46.31	42.97	41.69
	SD	23.73	26.34	26.41	26.45
	PRMT	48.93	44.29	27.39	23.75
HSAL-Sensory	SD	26.91	23.72	16.17	15.8
	Wilcoxon Z	−0.61	−1.91	−3.86	−3.94
	p	n.s.	n.s.	<0.001	<0.001
	CMT	19.3	20.52	19.59	18.69
	SD	9.64	10.61	11.4	10.36
	PRMT	23.29	20.46	12.25	10.32
BDI-II score	SD	11.58	10.7	7.62	5.9
	Wilcoxon Z	−0.6	−2.35	−4.21	−4.41
	p	n.s.	<0.05	<0.001	0.001
	CMT	39.9	39.73	39.09	38.52
	SD	14.1	16.23	16.86	16.42
	PRMT	38.26	36.12	25.95	23.82
ODI (%)	SD	12.5	14.06	10.49	11.6
	Wilcoxon Z	−0.09	−2.09	−4.19	−4.2
	p	n.s.	<0.05	<0.001	<0.001

BDI-II: Beck Depression Inventory, 2nd version; ODI: Oswestry Disability Index; PRMT: Psycho-regulatory massage therapy; CMT: classical massage therapy; n.s.: not significant.

ODI (%) score for disability: The progression of improvement in functional status achieved by PRMT in comparison to CMT is quite similar to that for depression. A weak, yet significantly better improvement in PRMT than in CMT occurred in T1, but much greater treatment differences appeared in T2 and T3. The Friedmann ANOVA showed non-significant change by CMT ($p = 0.56$). In contrast, there was a significant change in ODI (%) by PRMT ($p < 0.001$) with significant post hoc differences in all comparisons, except for T3 vs. T2. Table 4 shows the distribution of patients within the different levels of disability (reflecting limitations in quality of life, daily activities, and participation) at baseline and follow-up measurements. Before intervention, the vast majority (90.62%) of the PRMT group had a moderate to severe level of disability. At follow-up, 86.66% of the patients had minimal to moderate levels of disability. On average, the degree of disability improved by at least one level in 90% of the PRMT group, while CMT did not lead to any substantial change. The effect size according to Cohen, $f = 0.47$, corresponds to a strong effect.

Table 4. Distribution of patients at baseline (T0) and follow-up (T3) according to the respective levels of disability.

Level of Disability	PRMT n = 28		CMT n = 29	
	T0	T3	T0	T3
Minimal	6.25%	43.33%	9.09%	10.34%
Moderate	46.87%	43.33%	45.45%	51.73%
Severe	43.75%	13.34%	33.34%	20.69%
Crippled	3.12%	0%	12.12%	17.24%
Bedridden	0%	0%	0%	0%

4. Discussion

The primary aim of this study was to examine the effect of two forms of massage therapy in patients with chronic back pain (cBP). According to the general consensus about pain as a multidimensional experience [49,50] pain was assessed via HSAL (the Hamburg Pain Adjective List). In the group receiving PRMT, the decrease in the HSAL total score was statistically significant (−57.7 points), relating to an improvement of 46%. In contrast, the HSAL total score improved only by 5.6% in the group receiving CMT, failing to reach statistical significance and indicating no clinical relevance. In terms of decrease in symptoms of affective and sensory pain experience, PRMT thus shows strong superiority over CMT. Consistent with our results, Cherkin et al. [51] investigated 10 massage applications with a duration of 50–60 min and compared "structural" massages with relaxing massages. Relaxing massages were superior to structural massages, the latter being comparable to CMT. The follow-up at 10 weeks showed that the results persisted in both groups; thus, a long-term effect analogous to the results of the present study could also be observed. Without emphasizing different techniques, Wallach et al. [52] observed a sustained long-term effect of CMT after three months involving 10 applications of massage therapy of 20 min each over 10 weeks. Hamre et al. [53] investigated the effect of rhythmic massage therapy in a four-year prospective cohort study. They examined 85 chronically ill patients, 45 of whom suffered from chronic back or neck pain. Eighteen of the patients also suffered from depression and fatigue. The disease and symptom scores used in that study, each on a scale of 0 to 10, improved significantly. The disease score decreased from 6.3 to 2.77 points, and the symptom score decreased from 5.76 to 3.13 points. The SF-36 questionnaire also showed an improvement in the physical component score and the mental score. Thus, the symptoms of chronic disease were reduced, and at the same time, the quality of life of the patients improved.

Models from neuro-biological research might explain the positive effects of massage and the role of their specific techniques. Studies using microneurography have indicated the existence of low-threshold slowly conducting C-fibers in superficial skin layers that are predominantly activated by soft and low-velocity (3 cm/s) stroking stimuli [27]. In contrast, stronger pressure stimuli penetrating into deeper subepidermal skin layers activate rapidly conducting A-tactile afferents. A-tactile and C-tactile afferents are regarded as important for discriminant and affective dimensions of touch perception, respectively [28]. Accordingly, A-tactile fibers are predominantly abundant in the glabrous skin of the hands, whereas C-tactile fibers predominate in the hairy skin of the limbs and back. Several authors have pointed to the importance of the type of touch to be applied: slow, harmonic, and rhythmic with moderate pressure [24,54–57].

Boehme et al. compared patients suffering from fibromyalgia with healthy controls by using functional magnetic resonance imaging (fMRI) imaging of brain activity in response to selective C-tactile stimuli and additionally analyzed the voxel-based morphometry in areas of the limbic cortex [58]. They observed an abnormal pattern of deactivation and activation within the posterior insula during pleasantness and pain ratings, respectively, and a reduced grey matter density in the hippocampus and anterior insula. The authors interpreted their results as indications of anhedonia to gentle touch in fibromyalgia. Notably, classical massage is reported to worsen pain, whereas soft skin stroking, lymphatic drainage, and superficial vacuum massage alleviate pain in fibromyalgia patients [59]. Liljencrantz and Olausson [56] also reported anxiety-reducing effects of stimulating C-tactile afferents.

Craig [60] and Devue et al. [61] identified a functional network between the anterior insula and the cingulate gyrus, which serves primarily for self-recognition and awareness of one's own body. External impulses like touch and their subjective processing are thus integrated into emotional experiences. Older studies identified interoceptive afferents of primates as correlates of a so-called "gut feeling", which represents a complex integration of sensory perceptions and corresponding emotional responses. In the early 1990s, Damasio demonstrated that emotional and mental responses to stimuli mediate spino-thalamic and insular impulses that are integrated into body perception [62]. Paulsen and Stein reported that patients with depression and/or anxiety disorders experience significantly altered interoceptive signal processing. Signals are passed on blurred and amplified, so that homeostatic states are difficult to predict [63].

Several studies have shown an interaction of C-tactile afferents with the oxytonergic system in reducing pain and improving body perception [24,54,55]. Pfeifer et al. [64] and Uvnäs-Moberg and Peterson [23] postulated a positive influence on pain memory via the limbic system and activation of the oxytonergic system. This hypothesis was confirmed by follow-up data. A long-term effect was shown in both groups at three months post-intervention. This is coherent with the neuro-biologic findings by Lund et al. [65], who reported a long-term pain-reducing effect of soft massage-like touch through interaction of the oxytonergic system with the opioid system and activation of periaqueductal grey neurons. Miranda-Cardenaz et al. [66] and DeLaTorre [67] detected oxytocin receptors in the laminae of the dorsal horns. By micro-stimulation of the paraventricular nucleus and intrathecal administration of oxytocin, they were able to demonstrate an inhibited stimulus response of the wide dynamic-range neurons in the spinal horn in chronic pain syndrome. The authors considered this to be a descending oxytonergic control mechanism that influences chronic pain perception. Oxytocin also plays an antagonistic role in the glutamatergic spinal sensory conduction of acute pain stimuli [68]. Oxytocin inhibits the conduction of pain in the protopathic ascending pathways and plays a role in the function of the opioid system and gate control mechanism [64,65]. Thus, oxytocin can inhibit acute and chronic pain stimuli at different levels of the central nervous system (CNS).

The results on depression severity in our study, as measured by the BDI-II questionnaire, lend further strong support for the importance of C-tactile stimulation underlying the superior efficacy of PRMT over CMT. In the PRMT group, improvements on the BDI-II correspond to a moderate clinical effect [46]. In contrast, the severity of depression did not change significantly following CMT. These results support findings from a systematic review by Baumgart et al. that found massage therapy to be effective for depression and anxiety as a primary diagnosis and a co-morbidity, respectively [16]. Finally, disability and activity improved significantly within the PRMT group. Inter-group analysis also showed a significant effect in favor of PRMT compared to CMT. The PRMT group showed an improvement rate of 37.76%—the CMT group, only 3.46%. Changes of at least 18% are considered clinically relevant [46]. In this study, an important aim of chronic pain treatment (increase in function and activity) was achieved with PRMT [61]. Positive psycho-emotional effects, including a decrease in depressive symptoms, increase the motivation to maintain physical integrity, which is associated with an increase in personal activity [20,69,70]. Perceiving the back as a pleasant body part might reduce negative self-referential processing and open the patients towards treatments aiming at cognitive emotion regulation, e.g., mindfulness training [71].

There are limitations of our study. Since this study was conducted in the outpatient setting of a physiotherapy practice, the level of treatment standardization was low. Factors such as the patient's daily routine; sleep, waking, and eating rhythm; and time of intervention were not standardized to increase external validity. Treatment prescription was done by private orthopedic surgeons and general practitioners using the ICD-10 codes M54 and F45, which qualified the patients for study inclusion. There might have been variability among doctors in the use of these diagnoses. Yet, no patient had indication of specific back diseases causing their pain. Use of the term "somatoform" might be debatable, and it differs between the DSM (Diagnostic and Statistical Manual of Mental Disorders) and ICD classifications. During the update to DSM-5, the class of "somatoform disorders" was changed to "somatic symptom disorder", whereas the term is still used in the ICD-10. Furthermore, patients were allowed to use their pain medication as usual and receive other therapies, introducing a certain risk of bias to our results. Future studies could examine how the use of analgesics can be reduced by PRMT. Standard regulations of health care insurances allow 20 to 30 min of treatment duration for CMT, but 60 min for PRMT, because the latter involves a whole-body massage. Thus, longer treatment sessions might have contributed to the superiority of PRMT over CMT. The follow-up period of our study was three months, to increase comparability with other studies [16]. However, future studies could choose a longer follow-up period to better assess the long-term effects of PRMT intervention. Although the BDI-II score yielded no significant group differences at baseline, there was no stratification of patients according to the severity of depressive symptoms by an expert in psychiatry. Our results strongly suggest that patients with indications of depressive comorbidity benefit the most from PRMT. Although our a priori concept and conduct of PRMT aimed at an optimization of recruiting C-tactile afferent activity, we have no physiological proof of its importance in our study. Heart rate variability analysis has been found to be sensitive to the pleasantness of C-tactile stimulation [72] and appears to be compatible with study designs such as the one presented here.

5. Conclusions

Our results indicate that psycho-regulatory massage therapy (PRMT) is more effective than classical massage therapy (CMT) in reducing pain and depression and enhancing physical capacity and activity in patients suffering from chronic unspecific back pain. Unlike CMT, PRMT characterizes a massage technique by which the therapist applies soft and slow strokes upon the skin of the back, neck, shoulders, and upper arms that specifically activate C-tactile fibers. Future studies should examine the importance of individual differences of co-morbidity with depression in patients suffering from chronic unspecific back pain for the superiority of PRMT over CMT. This knowledge would improve the selection of individualized physical therapy options for these patients.

Author Contributions: S.B.-E.B.: Conceptualization, formal analysis, resources, writing—original draft. A.B.-K.: writing—review and editing, visualization. J.L.: Supervision, statistical analysis, writing—review and editing. All authors have read and agreed to the published version of the manuscript.

Funding: This research received no external funding.

Conflicts of Interest: The authors declare no conflict of interest.

References

1. Vos, T.; Barber, R.M.; Bell, B.; Bertozzi-Villa, A.; Biryukov, S.; Bolliger, I.; Charlson, F.; Davis, A.; Degenhardt, L.; Dicker, D.; et al. Global, regional, and national incidence, prevalence, and years lived with disability for 301 acute and chronic diseases and injuries in 188 countries, 1990–2013: A systematic analysis for the Global Burden of Disease Study 2013. *Lancet* **2015**, *386*, 743–800. [CrossRef]
2. Schneider, S.; Randoll, D.; Buchner, M. Why do women have back pain more than men? *Clin. J. Pain* **2006**, *22*, 738–747. [CrossRef] [PubMed]
3. Van Middelkoop, M.; Rubinstein, S.M.; Kuijpers, T.; Verhagen, A.P.; Ostelo, R.W.; Koes, B.W.; van Tulder, M. A systematic review on the effectiveness of physical and rehabilitation interventions for chronic non-specific low back pain. *Eur. Spine J.* **2010**, *20*, 19–39. [CrossRef] [PubMed]
4. Khadilkar, A.; Milne, S.; Brosseau, L.; Wells, G.; Tugwell, P.; Robinson, V.; Shea, B.; Saginur, M. Transcutaneous electrical nerve stimulation for the treatment of chronic low back pain: A systematic review. *Spine* **2005**, *30*, 2657–2666. [CrossRef] [PubMed]
5. Xu, M.; Yan, S.; Yin, X.; Li, X.; Gao, S.; Han, R.; Wei, L.; Luo, W.; Lei, G. Acupuncture for chronic low back pain in long-term follow-up: A meta-analysis of 13 randomized controlled trials. *Am. J. Chin. Med.* **2013**, *41*, 1–19. [CrossRef]

6. Glazov, G.; Yelland, M.; Emery, J. Low-level laser therapy for chronic non-specific low back pain: A meta-analysis of randomised controlled trials. *Acupunct. Med.* **2016**, *34*, 328–341. [CrossRef] [PubMed]
7. Seco-Calvo, J.; Kovacs, F.M.; Urrútia, G. The efficacy, safety, effectiveness, and cost-effectiveness of ultrasound and shock wave therapies for low back pain: A systematic review. *Spine J.* **2011**, *11*, 966–977. [CrossRef]
8. Oliveira, C.B.; Maher, C.G.; Pinto, R.Z.; Traeger, A.C.; Lin, C.-W.C.; Chenot, J.-F.; van Tulder, M.; Koes, B.W. Clinical practice guidelines for the management of non-specific low back pain in primary care: An updated overview. *Eur. Spine J.* **2018**, *27*, 2791–2803. [CrossRef]
9. Airaksinen, O.; Brox, J.I.; Cedraschi, C.; Hildebrandt, J.; Klaber-Moffett, J.; Kovacs, F.; Mannion, A.F.; Reis, S.; Staal, J.B.; Ursin, H.; et al. Chapter 4 European guidelines for the management of chronic nonspecific low back pain. *Eur. Spine J.* **2006**, *15*, 192–300. [CrossRef]
10. Chou, R. Nonpharmacologic therapies for low back pain. *Ann. Intern. Med.* **2017**, *167*, 606–607. [CrossRef]
11. Levenig, C.G.; Kellmann, M.; Kleinert, J.; Belz, J.; Hesselmann, T.; Hasenbring, M.I. Body image is more negative in patients with chronic low back pain than in patients with subacute low back pain and healthy controls. *Scand. J. Pain* **2019**, *19*, 147–156. [CrossRef] [PubMed]
12. Rohricht, F.; Beyer, W.; Priebe, S. Disturbances of body-experience in acute anxiety and depressive disorders neuroticism or somatization? *Psychother. Psych. Med.* **2002**, *52*, 205–213.
13. Field, T. Massage therapy. *Med. Clin. North Am.* **2002**, *86*, 163–171. [CrossRef]
14. Baumgart, S. Psychoaktive massage und atemtherapie-konzept und fallbericht. *Phys. Ther. Theor. Prax.* **2008**, *6*, 277–281.
15. Dogs, W. Psychomotorik der massage. *Phys. Ther.* **1988**, *1*, 12–14.
16. Baumgart, S.; Müller-Oerlinghausen, B.; Schendera, C.F.G. Wirksamkeit der massagetherapie bei depression und angsterkrankungen sowie bei depressivität und angst als komorbidität—eine systematische übersicht kontrollierter studien. *Phys. Med. Rehabil. Kurortmed.* **2011**, *21*, 167–182. [CrossRef]
17. Müller-Oerlinghausen, B.; Berg, C.; Droll, W. Die Slow Stroke®massage als ein körpertherapeutischer ansatz bei depression. *Psychiatr. Prax.* **2007**, *34*, 305–308. [CrossRef]
18. Listing, M.; Reißhauer, A.; Krohn, M.; Voigt, B.; Tjahono, G.; Becker, J.; Klapp, B.F.; Rauchfuß, M. Massage therapy reduces physical discomfort and improves mood disturbances in women with breast cancer. *Psychol. Oncol.* **2009**, *18*, 1290–1299. [CrossRef]
19. Diego, M.A.; Field, T.; Sanders, C.; Hernandez-Reif, M. Massage therapy of moderate and light pressure and vibration effects on EEG and heart rate. *Int. J. Neurosci.* **2004**, *114*, 31–44. [CrossRef]
20. Olausson, H.W.; Wessberg, J.; Morrison, I.; McGlone, F.; Vallbo, Å. The neurophysiology of unmyelinated tactile afferents. *Neurosci. Biobehav. Rev.* **2010**, *34*, 185–191. [CrossRef]
21. Moyer, C.A. Massage therapy: An examination of the contextual model. *Diss. Abstr. Int. Sect. B Sci. Eng.* **2008**, *69*, 1337.
22. Kolster, B.C. Wirkprinzipien der massage. In *Massage*; Springer: Berlin/Heidelberg, Germany, 2003; pp. 22–34.
23. Uvnas-Moberg, K.; Petersson, M. Oxytocin, a mediator of anti-stress, well-being, social interaction, growth and healing. *Z Psychosom. Med. Psychother.* **2005**, *51*, 57–80. [PubMed]
24. Walker, S.C.; McGlone, F.P. The social brain: Neurobiological basis of affiliative behaviours and psychological well-being. *Neuropeptides* **2013**, *47*, 379–393. [CrossRef] [PubMed]
25. McGlone, F.; Wessberg, J.; Olausson, H. Discriminative and affective touch: Sensing and feeling. *Neuron* **2014**, *82*, 737–755. [CrossRef] [PubMed]
26. Kain, K.L.; Levine, P.A.; Terrell, S.J. *Nurturing Resilience: Helping Clients Move Forward from Developmental Trauma*; North Atlantic Books: Berkeley, CA, USA, 2018.
27. Shaikh, S.; Nagi, S.S.; McGlone, F.; Mahns, D.A. Psychophysical Investigations into the role of low-threshold C fibres in non-painful affective processing and pain modulation. *PLoS ONE* **2015**, *10*, e0138299. [CrossRef] [PubMed]
28. Okabe, S.; Yoshida, M.; Takayanagi, Y.; Onaka, T. Activation of hypothalamic oxytocin neurons following tactile stimuli in rats. *Neurosci. Lett.* **2015**, *600*, 22–27. [CrossRef] [PubMed]
29. Richard, P.; Moos, F.; Freund-Mercier, M.J. Central effects of oxytocin. *Physiol. Rev.* **1991**, *71*, 331–370. [CrossRef]
30. Dworkin, R.H.; Turk, D.C.; Peirce-Sandner, S.; Baron, R.; Bellamy, N.; Burke, L.B.; Chappell, A.; Chartier, K.; Cleeland, C.S.; Costello, A.; et al. Research design considerations for confirmatory chronic pain clinical trials: IMMPACT recommendations. *Pain* **2010**, *149*, 177–193. [CrossRef]

31. Henningsen, P. The psychosomatics of chronic back pain. Classification, aetiology and therapy. *Orthopäde* **2004**, *33*, 558–567. [CrossRef]
32. Abraham, I.; Killackey-Jones, B. Lack of evidence-based research for idiopathic low back pain. *Arch. Intern. Med.* **2002**, *162*, 1442–1444. [CrossRef]
33. Deyo, R.A. Diagnostic Evaluation of LBP. *Arch. Intern. Med.* **2002**, *162*, 1444–1447. [CrossRef] [PubMed]
34. Dworkin, R.H.; Turk, D.C.; Wyrwich, K.W.; Beaton, D.; Cleeland, C.S.; Farrar, J.T.; Haythornthwaite, J.A.; Jensen, M.P.; Kerns, R.D.; Ader, D.N.; et al. Interpreting the clinical importance of treatment outcomes in chronic pain clinical trials: Immpact recommendations. *J. Pain* **2008**, *9*, 105–121. [CrossRef] [PubMed]
35. Moyer, C.A.; Rounds, J.; Hannum, J.W. A meta-analysis of massage therapy research. *Psychol. Bull.* **2004**, *130*, 3–18. [CrossRef]
36. Sherman, K.J.; Cook, A.J.; Wellman, R.D.; Hawkes, R.J.; Kahn, J.R.; Deyo, R.A.; Cherkin, D.C. Five-week outcomes from a dosing trial of therapeutic massage for chronic neck pain. *Ann. Fam. Med.* **2014**, *12*, 112–120. [CrossRef] [PubMed]
37. Hoppe, F. *Hamburger Schmerz-Adjektiv-Liste (HSAL)*; Beltz: Weinheim, Germany, 1991.
38. Lehrl, S.; Cziske, R.; Blaha, L. *Schmerzmessung Durch die Mehr Dimensionale Schmerzskala—MSS*; Vless GmbH: Munich, Germany, 1980.
39. Laux, L.; Glanzmann, P.; Schaffner, P.; Spielberger, C.D. *Das State-Trait-Angstinventar. Theoretische Grundlagen und Handanweisung*; State Trait Anxiety Inventory. Theoretical Foundations and Manual; Beltz: Weinheim, Germany, 1981.
40. Hautzinger, M.; Keller, F.; Kühner, C. *BDI-II Beck-Depressions-Inventar Revision*, 2nd ed.; Pearson Assessment: Frankfurt, Germany, 2009.
41. Beck, A.T.; Steer, R.A.; Brown, G.K. Manual for the beck depression inventory-II. San Antonio. *TX Psychol. Corp.* **1996**, *1*, 82.
42. Hiroe, T.; Kojima, M.; Yamamoto, I.; Nojima, S.; Kinoshita, Y.; Hashimoto, N.; Watanabe, N.; Maeda, T.; Furukawa, T.A. Gradations of clinical severity and sensitivity to change assessed with the Beck Depression Inventory-II in Japanese patients with depression. *Psychiatry Res.* **2005**, *135*, 229–235. [CrossRef]
43. Fairbank, J.C.; Couper, J.; Davies, J.B.; O'Brien, J.P. The Oswestry low back pain disability questionnaire. *Physiotherapy* **1980**, *66*, 271–273.
44. Mannion, A.F.; Junge, A.; Fairbank, J.C.T.; Dvořák, J.; Grob, D. Development of a German version of the Oswestry Disability Index. Part 1: Cross-cultural adaptation, reliability, and validity. *Eur. Spine J.* **2005**, *15*, 55–65. [CrossRef]
45. Mannion, A.F.; Junge, A.; Grob, D.; Dvořák, J.; Fairbank, J.C.T. Development of a German version of the Oswestry Disability Index. Part 2: Sensitivity to change after spinal surgery. *Eur. Spine J.* **2005**, *15*, 66–73. [CrossRef]
46. Van Hooff, M.L.; Spruit, M.; Fairbank, J.C.T.; van Limbeek, J.; Wilco, J.C.H. The Oswestry Disability Index (version 2.1 a): Validation of a Dutch language version. *Spine* **2015**, *40*, 83–90. [CrossRef]
47. Fairbank, J.C.T.; Pynsent, P.B. The Oswestry Disability Index. *Spine* **2000**, *25*, 2940–2953. [CrossRef] [PubMed]
48. Tal-Akabi, A.; Oesch, P. Behinderung bei rückenbeschwerden: Oswestry Disability questionnaire—Deutsche version (ODI-D.). In *Assessments in der Rehabilitation*, 2nd ed.; Oesch, P., Hilfiker, R., Keller, S., Kool, J., Luomajoki, H., Schädler, S., Tal-Akabi, A., Verra, M., Leu, C.W., Eds.; Verlag Hans Huber: Bern, Switzerland, 2011; Volume 2, pp. 296–300.
49. Dworkin, R.H.; Turk, D.C.; Farrar, J.T.; Haythornthwaite, J.A.; Jensen, M.P.; Katz, N.P.; Kerns, R.D.; Stucki, G.; Allen, R.R.; Bellamy, N.; et al. Core outcome measures for chronic pain clinical trials: IMMPACT recommendations. *Pain* **2005**, *113*, 9–19. [CrossRef] [PubMed]
50. Boonstra, A.M.; Preuper, H.R.S.; Reneman, M.F.; Posthumus, J.B.; Stewart, R.E. Reliability and validity of the visual analogue scale for disability in patients with chronic musculoskeletal pain. *Int. J. Rehabil. Res.* **2008**, *31*, 165–169. [CrossRef]
51. Cherkin, D.C.; Sherman, K.J.; Kahn, J.; Wellman, M.R.; Cook, A.J.; Johnson, M.E.; Erro, R.J.; Delaney, M.K.; Deyo, R.A. A comparison of the effects of 2 types of massage and usual care on chronic low back pain. *Ann. Intern. Med.* **2011**, *155*. [CrossRef]
52. Walach, H.; Güthlin, C.; König, M. Efficacy of massage therapy in chronic pain: A pragmatic randomized trial. *J. Altern. Complement. Med.* **2003**, *9*, 837–846. [CrossRef]

53. Hamre, H.J.; Witt, C.M.; Glockmann, A.; Ziegler, R.; Willich, S.N.; Kiene, H. Rhythmical massage therapy in chronic disease: A 4-year prospective cohort study. *J. Altern. Complement. Med.* **2007**, *13*, 635–642. [CrossRef] [PubMed]
54. Lloyd, D.M.; McGlone, F.P.; Yosipovitch, G. Somatosensory pleasure circuit: From skin to brain and back. *Exp. Dermatol.* **2015**, *24*, 321–324. [CrossRef] [PubMed]
55. Krahé, C.; Drabek, M.M.; Paloyelis, Y.; Fotopoulou, A. Affective touch and attachment style modulate pain: A laser-evoked potentials study. *Philos. Trans. R. Soc. B Biol. Sci.* **2016**, *371*, 20160009. [CrossRef]
56. Liljencrantz, J.; Olausson, H. Tactile C fibers and their contributions to pleasant sensations and to tactile allodynia. *Front. Behav. Neurosci.* **2014**, *8*, 37. [CrossRef]
57. Kaplan, C. An Examination of Brain Network Organization and the Analgesic Mechanisms of a Non-Pharmacological Treatment in Chronic Centralized Pain. Ph.D. Thesis, University of Michigan, Ann Arbor, MI, USA, 2018.
58. Boehme, R.; van Ettinger-Veenstra, H.; Olausson, H.; Gerdle, B.; Nagi, S.S. Anhedonia to gentle touch in fibromyalgia: Normal sensory processing but abnormal evaluation. *Brain Sci.* **2020**, *10*, 306. [CrossRef] [PubMed]
59. Weiss, T. Fibromyalgie-ein chronisch-generalisierendes Sensitivierungssyndrom? *PiD Psychother. im Dialog* **2005**, *6*, 59–65. [CrossRef]
60. Craig, A.D. How do you feel—now? The anterior insula and human awareness. *Nat. Rev. Neurosci.* **2009**, *10*, 59–70. [CrossRef] [PubMed]
61. Devue, C.; Collette, F.; Balteau, E.; Degueldre, C.; Luxen, A.; Maquet, P.; Brédart, S. Here I am: The cortical correlates of visual self-recognition. *Brain Res.* **2007**, *1143*, 169–182. [CrossRef]
62. Damasio, A.R. *Descartes' Error: Emotion, Reason and the Human Brain*; Putnam: New York, NY, USA, 1994.
63. Paulus, M.P.; Stein, M.B. Interoception in anxiety and depression. *Brain Struct. Funct.* **2010**, *214*, 451–463. [CrossRef]
64. Pfeifer, A.-C.; Ditzen, B.; Neubauer, E.; Schiltenwolf, M. Wirkung von Oxytocin auf das menschliche Schmerzerleben Effect of oxytocin on human pain perception. *Schmerz* **2016**, *30*, 457–469. [CrossRef]
65. Lund, I.; Yu, L.C.; Uvnäs-Moberg, K.; Wang, J.; Yu, C.; Kurosawa, M.; Agren, G.; Rosen, A.; Lekman, M.; Lundeberg, T. Repeated massage-like stimulation induces long term effects on nociception: Contribution of oxytonergic mechanisms. *Eur. J. Neurosci.* **2005**, *22*, 1553–1554. [CrossRef]
66. Miranda-Cardenas, Y.; Rojas-Piloni, G.; Martínez-Lorenzana, G.; Rodríguez-Jiménez, J.; López-Hidalgo, M.; Freund-Mercier, M.J.; Condés-Lara, M. Oxytocin and electrical stimulation of the paraventricular hypothalamic nucleus produce antinociceptive effects that are reversed by an oxytocin antagonist. *Pain* **2006**, *122*, 182–189. [CrossRef]
67. DeLaTorre, S.; Rojas-Piloni, G.; Martinez-Lorenzana, G.J.; Villanueva, L.; Rodrigues-Jimenez, J.; Villanueva, L.; Condes-Lara, M. Paraventricular oxitocinergic hypothalamic prevention or interruption of long-term potentiation in dorsal horn nociceptive neurons: Electrophysiological and behavioral evidence. *Pain* **2009**, *144*, 320–328. [CrossRef] [PubMed]
68. Jo, Y.H.; Stoeckel, M.E.; Freund-Mercier, M.J.; Schlichter, R. Oxytocin modulates glutamatergic synaptic transmission between cultured neonatal spinal cord dorsal horn neurons. *J. Neurosci.* **1998**, *18*, 2377–2386. [CrossRef]
69. Sprott, H. Pathophysiologie der peripheren Schmerzentstehung–therapeutische Angriffspunkte. *Praxis* **2016**, *105*, 1267–1271. [CrossRef]
70. Schleip, R.; Jäger, H. *Lehrbuch Faszien: Grundlagen, Forschung, Behandlung*; Urban & Fischer: Munich, Germany, 2014; pp. 65–68.
71. Chiesa, A.; Serretti, A.; Jakobsen, J.C. Mindfulness: Top–down or bottom–up emotion regulation strategy? *Clin. Psychol. Rev.* **2013**, *33*, 82–96. [CrossRef] [PubMed]
72. Triscoli, C.; Croy, I.; Steudte-Schmiedgen, S.; Olausson, H.; Sailer, U. Heart rate variability is enhanced by long-lasting pleasant touch at CT-optimized velocity. *Biol. Psychol.* **2017**, *128*, 71–81. [CrossRef] [PubMed]

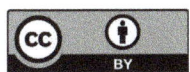

© 2020 by the authors. Licensee MDPI, Basel, Switzerland. This article is an open access article distributed under the terms and conditions of the Creative Commons Attribution (CC BY) license (http://creativecommons.org/licenses/by/4.0/).

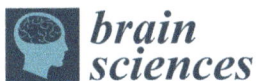

Review

Keeping in Touch with Mental Health: The Orienting Reflex and Behavioral Outcomes from Calatonia

Anita Ribeiro Blanchard [1],* and William Edgar Comfort [2]

1. Faculty of Psychology, University of Barcelona, 08035 Barcelona, Spain
2. Social and Cognitive Science Laboratory, Centre for Health and Biological Sciences, Mackenzie Presbyterian University, São Paulo 01241, Brazil; 9032936@mackenzie.br
* Correspondence: aribeiri8@alumnes.ub.edu

Received: 8 February 2020; Accepted: 20 March 2020; Published: 22 March 2020

Abstract: Physical and psychological therapy based on touch has been gradually integrated into broader mental health settings in the past two decades, evolving from a variety of psychodynamic, neurobiological and trauma-based approaches, as well as Eastern and spiritual philosophies and other integrative and converging systems. Nevertheless, with the exception of a limited number of well-known massage therapy techniques, only a few structured protocols of touch therapy have been standardized and researched to date. This article describes a well-defined protocol of touch therapy in the context of psychotherapy—the Calatonia technique—which engages the orienting reflex. The orienting reflex hypothesis is explored here as one of the elements of this technique that helps to decrease states of hypervigilance and chronic startle reactivity (startle and defensive reflexes) and restore positive motivational and appetitive states.

Keywords: orienting reflex; motivational system; touch therapy; integrative psychotherapy; somatic psychology

1. Introduction

The limitations of verbal psychotherapy have become more evident in the past thirty years [1], giving rise to a large number of somatic and body-based modalities aimed to address treatment-resistant disorders [2–4]. Recently, there has been an interest in developing somatically informed research methods to support a wide range of these integrative practices [5,6]. Accordingly, this article discusses the significance of integrating a structured touch therapy (Calatonia) into psychotherapy to facilitate an orienting reflex (OR) [7]. The OR leads the individual to direct their motivational system towards appetitive and exploratory states, which can, in turn, positively influence affective and cognitive states.

Motivation—a concept derived from the biological sciences—has not been explored for its potential strength in mental health treatments, although motivation as a cognitive concept was well developed by Miller [8]. Affective responses comprising an organism's underlying motivational state have been broadly categorized in terms of defensive and appetitive systems, evolving either separately or in conjunction to engage with environmental stimuli indicative of threat or opportunities for survival, respectively [9]. In this perspective, emotional experiences occur within a range of appetitive-pleasant or defensive-unpleasant valence and have levels of arousal that indicate the degree of activation in response to that emotional valence [10]. These two basic dimensions of affective responses support mobilization for action, attention and social communication, according to the motivational system that is engaged (defensive or appetitive), its intensity of activation and its emotional context [9–13].

While several findings have identified distinct brain networks for approach/avoidance behavior and pleasant or aversive affect in healthy subjects [14,15], mental health continues to be studied primarily from a symptomatological perspective, with little research into long-term behavioral outcomes linked to the patient's motivational state.

As an illustration, depressive disorders—from their biological symptoms to their emotional and cognitive expression—can be understood as dysfunctions of the motivational system, in which (appetitive) motivation is reduced. Anxiety disorders may also be viewed from a motivational system perspective, in which there is either strong behavioral inhibition or impulsivity, based on aversive, defensive or avoidant motivation [16]. In such cases, touch therapies may prove useful to redirect the individual's motivational state toward more approach-oriented behavior, in conjunction with conventional psychotherapy and/or pharmacological treatment.

It is in this context that we introduce the therapeutic potential of Calatonia, a long-standing technique of touch therapy which aims to re-orient the individual toward a more open behavioral approach through activation of the appetitive motivational system and concomitant inhibition of startle and defensive states. This integrative approach has been used to treat disorders unresponsive to verbal psychotherapy alone, such as PTSD and other forms of trauma.

The primary mechanism through which Calatonia is thought to exert changes in the individual's motivational states is by eliciting an orienting reflex (OR) within the context of psychotherapy [17]. The OR is activated through touch experienced as a novel, sustained and non-threatening stimulus. Calatonia (described in Section 3) is a therapeutic technique based on a structured sequence of touches applied bilaterally to distinct regions of the body [18–20]. Since its inception, Calatonia has purported to induce a state of deep relaxation and increased unconscious processing with a net result of altering the patient's motivational and affective states [19–21].

However, Calatonia has yet to be submitted to rigorous scientific testing for the direct therapeutic benefits accrued from its application. One potential avenue for such research is the Research Domain Criteria (RDoC) framework for evaluating novel treatments for mental health put forth by the National Institute of Mental Health (NIMH) [22]. Within the RDoC framework, an upward level of analysis constitutes mapping functional measures of neural activity to variation in clinical symptoms on a distinct spectrum of mental health such as anxiety [22]. In line with this approach, a study utilizing near-infrared spectroscopy (fNIRS) to investigate alterations in neural markers of anxiety following Calatonia is currently under preparation.

2. History of the Technique

During WWII, the Hungarian physician Pethö Sándor (1916–1992) structured a sequence of ten light touches while treating the psychological and physical suffering of refugees and other displaced persons at Red Cross refugee camps. This sequence of touches emerged from the combined biomedical knowledge and feedback from patients about the points of tactile contact that appeared to balance their sympathetic and parasympathetic responses and foster autonomic regulation [18–20].

After being treated with this technique—then named Calatonia—patients spontaneously shared their feelings, thoughts, worries, memories and traumatic experiences with a scale of trust and openness that had not happened before the treatment—a clear validation of its usefulness in psychotherapy [19,20]. Following a few applications of Calatonia, patients showed decreased symptoms of traumatic stress (shell shock), anxiety, depression, pain and other ailments that afflicted most war survivors at the time. Patients' improvements manifested in terms of increased morale, acceptance, well-being, hope, will to live, overall motivation and resilience [21], defined as the ability to adequately adapt and respond to homeostatic disturbances [23]. These touches seemed to promote global changes, which led Sándor [19,20] to describe Calatonia as a technique for psychophysical regulation and reorganization.

After the end of the war, Sándor worked for two years in the psychiatric wards of German hospitals, using Calatonia to successfully treat depression, suicide ideation, post-traumatic stress disorder, anxiety, catatonic states and other mental disorders [18,21,24,25]. Later, in São Paulo, Brazil [26], he expanded the repertoire of techniques to include many other "light touch" sequences, grouped under the name subtle touch (ST) [27–30]. Another ST technique, Fractional Decompression, works by gradually releasing pressure from a touch applied to hairy skin on the back, arms or legs [27]. Fractional decompression is thought to primarily target the affective-affiliative touch system associated with hairy non-glabrous skin [31]. Calatonia continues to be the most widely used ST technique. At times, subtle touch and Calatonia are used interchangeably to denote the whole gamut of techniques developed by Sándor and subsequently expanded by other clinical psychologists [32]. Sándor's subtle touch method has produced numerous qualitative studies published over the past four decades (reviewed in [32]), as well as quantitative research in the past fifteen years [32–34].

Sándor had previously hypothesized [19,20] that the experience of physiological regulation, mood stabilization, inflow of adaptive cognition and neuromuscular relaxation induced by Calatonia were linked to the associative activation of somatosensory representations in the frontotemporal cortex, the engagement of peripheral proprioceptive nerve fibers, particularly in the skin and cortical mediation by the ascending reticular activating system. Furthermore, he associated its effects with psycho-affective elements mobilized by the configuration of dyadic regulation through the touch therapy protocol.

Given the barriers to many forms of social and affiliative touch in social interactions, particularly in the context of psychotherapy, it can be useful to compare the touch sequence employed in Calatonia with other common forms of "pleasant" touch found in everyday encounters. In particular, a recently discovered category of slow-response unmyelinated nerve fiber, C-tactile afferents, have been implicated in many forms of innocuous touch [35], as well as touch in social contexts [31]. C-tactile afferent projections terminate in the ventral medial nucleus of the thalamus and posterior insular cortex [36,37], associated with the contextual and affective components of touch [38]. While the primary areas of contact in Calatonia are to the glabrous skin areas of the feet or hands (see below), the sequence employed also includes contact to hairy skin containing C-tactile afferent connections. Several other ST techniques similarly activate CT connections by contact with the arms, calves, back and head. As such, Calatonia may act on both a common affiliative system for social touch as well as on more discriminative neural pathways in glabrous areas of the hands and feet. However, the perceptual characteristics of touch in these regions are specifically modulated in Calatonia to induce large-scale novelty-related activation in addition to more familiar responses to CT touch primarily in thalamic and insular regions.

3. The Calatonia Technique

Touch therapies differ in their goals. Some focus on achieving body awareness, structural readjustment, functional improvement, emotional-affective regulation, release of pent up energy, healing of trauma, among other issues [2]. Calatonia has an open-ended goal, in contrast to more narrowly defined ST techniques: one geared toward spontaneous adaptive adjustments in one's idiosyncratic psychophysical needs and imbalances, prompted by the sequence of touches. As an example, for some, stress will manifest as insomnia or excessive worrying; for others, it will manifest as addiction, overeating or overreacting emotionally in relationships. Each maladaptive style will lead to different responses to Calatonia's applications, despite being caused by the same underlying problem—stress.

A description of this technique (Figures 1–5) may be useful to integrate the elements that will be discussed in this article. Calatonia is performed in silence (unless the patient feels discomfort or the need to speak) after the patient has been briefed on the steps of the protocol [19,20]. The patient removes his or her shoes and socks and lies on a massage table in a supine position, with his or her eyes closed, fully dressed (Figure 1). Preferably, the therapist applies the technique on the lower limbs, or, alternatively, on the hands and forearms. Excluding the tenth point (the head), the first nine points of tactile contact are bilateral (the same tactile stimulus is simultaneously held on each side of the body). The seven first touches (Figure 2) are extremely light (as if the therapist were holding a "soap bubble") and sustained in place for one to three minutes (preferably three minutes on the few initial applications). The eighth, ninth and tenth tactile contacts (respectively Figures 3–5) are supported and held in place for one to three minutes on the heels, calves and head (in that order). At the end, patients are coached back to awareness of the environment and themselves and instructed to sit up and walk back to their seat, at which point they are invited to share their observations or impressions, if any, which may have manifested during or after the application of the technique.

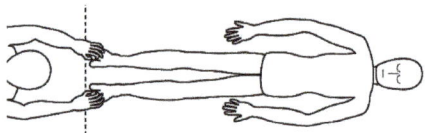

Figure 1. Resting state (task-free) supine position.

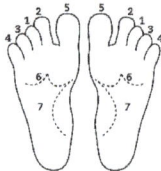

Figure 2. Sequential order of bilateral points of tactile contact.

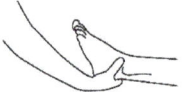

Figure 3. Ankle support, eighth bilateral touch.

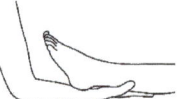

Figure 4. Calf support, ninth bilateral touch.

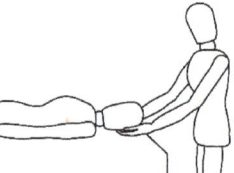

Figure 5. Head support, tenth and last touch.

4. Touch to the Feet or Hands

While it appears unusual to propose tactile contact with the patient's feet or hands in psychotherapy, there is strong empirical support for doing so. Contact is made to these specific sites, as nowhere else on the body is there found a similar configuration of neurobiological and physiological variables, including the distinctive dermo-mechanical features and receptors found on the glabrous skin of the feet and hands [35–44]. This combination of features frequently results in the activation of an orienting response by eliciting a pattern of neural activation associated with novelty, of either a neutral or pleasant nature, through both conscious and unconscious perceptual pathways.

The glabrous (non-hairy) skin of the hands and feet is indirectly connected to several perceptual subsystems involved in the detection of vibration, temperature changes and differences in texture and pressure, as well as somatosensory and proprioceptive responses [43,44]. The areas targeted in Calatonia contain the most numerous populations of skin receptors, collectively known as the discriminative–spatial system [41–46], distinct from receptors of the affective–affiliative system found primarily in non-glabrous skin. Glabrous skin is a dedicated site of very precise tactile perception geared toward the exploration of and adaptation to novel stimuli, as well as the evaluation and appraisal of a spectrum of touch pleasantness and roughness mediated by the somatosensory cortex [47–49].

For example, to read and attribute meaning to the raised dots of the Braille system requires language, touch and spatial coding to be transformed into semantic, lexical and haptic processing. This in turn engages highly associative areas of the brain to produce concrete and abstract thinking, symbols and ultimately communication [50].

Hands are also especially involved in the formation of procedural memory, which makes them potential "roads" for the emotional retrieval of such implicit memories—in particular, early childhood memories linked to independence, mastery, self-care, reaching out and so forth. These memories may be accompanied by emotional and relational contexts of frustration, impatience, among many other emotions and behavioral patterns [51,52]. Similarly, the locomotor system is in many ways involved in early childhood developmental milestones (standing, walking, running, bike riding, etc.).

The feet bear the total gravitational force imposed on the body and function as an integrated system with the cerebellum and vestibular system to control posture, coordination, equilibrium and the generation of locomotor rhythm; the proprioceptive control of posture is chiefly initiated in the feet [53]. Drew, Prentice and Schepens [54] state that these essential mechanisms of control of postural muscle tone and locomotion "are located in the brainstem and spinal cord, in which a range of locomotor behaviors are achieved by the projections from the forebrain structures (cerebral cortex, basal ganglia and limbic-hypothalamic systems) and cerebellum to the brainstem-spinal cord". As such, despite the role of these mechanisms in voluntary movement and locomotion, a significant portion of the adjustment of balance is made involuntarily, based on information that does not require conscious attention to be processed. When the feet are in an unloaded position (i.e., lying down), there is no background discharge activity in any of the cutaneous receptors unless there is intentionally applied stimulation [49,53–55]. This may be indicative of how Calatonia on the feet facilitates the reorganization of the individual's global posture and muscle tension.

5. Novel Stimuli in Psychotherapy

There are several common elements to Sándor's many ST techniques, yet two elements can be immediately perceived as fundamental: (a) their non-invasiveness, by respecting an individual's boundaries and even their resistance to therapy, while gently supporting the individual towards gaining resilience toward the integration of crucial personal issues; (b) their novelty, through the application of atypical sensory stimuli—not merely an oddball protocol for the sake of novelty itself, but a meaningful stimulus that engages global responses and multidimensional aspects of a person's life.

The combination of these two aspects, non-invasiveness and novelty, is hypothesized as generating an orienting reflex or an orienting response [7], also known as the 'what is it response?' or the exploratory response. The OR is an involuntary response of an organism to a stimulus that is 'out of the ordinary' but not alarming or menacing. ORs are an adaptive feature of cognition present since infancy [56] that play a major role in many aspects of motivation, emotion and attention [57–62].

Sándor purposefully developed different methods for creating ORs by using an unusually light and static form of touch or other forms of stimulation in his techniques. These included passive movements that were mechanically impossible for the patient to perform voluntarily (e.g., rotating the patient's finger sideways); atypical but non-threatening sounds directed towards specific parts of the body, small vibrations applied to bone projections and protuberances, such as the spinous processes [27] and many others. His approach was geared toward the enhancement of neural plasticity and the generation of 'dedicated neural circuitries' for experiencing well-being, leading to increased self-confidence and a sense of safety within one's own body [17,18].

6. The Orienting Reflex in Calatonia

An orienting reflex is triggered when a sensory stimulus is perceived as novel, innocuous or pleasant [58,63]. This may be seen in opposition to defensive reflexes initiated when a sensory stimulus is perceived as painful, aversive and potentially dangerous—or startle reflexes activated in response to abrupt, unexpected or overly intense stimuli. All of these responses, whether defensive/startle or orienting, will activate the executive network for regulation or action if necessary [64,65].

In animals, the OR is a survival reflex that does not burden the organism with a full-blown alert response but entices them to explore the environment. Pavlov [66] saw the OR as the biological basis for the highest form of curiosity, imagination, science and knowledge of the world around us. At the basic end of this spectrum, the OR encourages human curiosity, which drives child development and "involves an indissoluble mixture of cognition and motivation" [67]—a key prerequisite for learning and the formation of top-down predictions in perceptual processing. To achieve this level of exploration, the OR tunes the organism toward a specific stimulus by enhancing perceptual awareness [68–70]. In contrast, the defensive and startle reflexes limit the impact of the stimulus on the organism by functionally raising perceptual thresholds [68–70].

The OR halts all non-essential brain activity to allow the individual to orientate their primary senses towards the source of stimulation, focusing on possible means of interaction with the stimulus through the activation of the autonomic nervous system (ANS) [68,69]. It produces an unintentional shift of attention that interrupts the ordinary flow of awareness and leads us to attend to the novelty of a stimulus for the appraisal of its meaning and/or significance. This phase of the reflex has been classified by researchers as an "information-gathering", "analyzing", "modelling" or simply "sensory" phase [7]. One of the key physiological markers of an OR is the initial deceleration in the heartbeat, which is a sign of enhanced perceptual processing and is mediated by the parasympathetic branch of the ANS [71,72]. This initial slowdown allows the organism to more easily detect the potential significance of stimulus features to estimate 'uncertainty'. An OR is triggered if uncertainty is detected concerning the biological value or perceptual features of the stimulus [73].

As mentioned above, Calatonia triggers an OR due to its non-invasive nature (experienced as either of a neutral or pleasant affect), extended duration of passive tactile stimuli and the novelty of its touch. Sustained attention to a body location results in the enhanced processing of the tactile stimuli presented at that location compared to other unattended locations [74]. A light touch is often a strange sensory perception, particularly on the feet, accustomed to supporting the individual's body weight and rough contact with stimuli on the ground. The palms of the hands and the soles of the feet are instruments of self-agency [75–77] and rarely the object of passive interaction. Receiving a passive gentle touch in these areas may easily throw the organism into a state of perceptive, emotional and cognitive surprise yet still feel innocuous within a safe context. The neutral affect associated with the surprise response works to reset attentional processes [78]—with attention defined in cognitive terms as the ability to selectively attend to some stimuli while ignoring others [79].

Individuals have different forms of appraisal and emotional responses to touch based on their personal history and cultural biases [80]. However, it is highly likely that most people will experience an OR in response to an unexpectedly static, sustained and light touch that conveys neither personal meaning nor affection. Such a response is dependent on the therapist adopting an appropriately responsive but neutral affective state during the application of Calatonia.

7. Brain Areas Associated with the Orienting Reflex

Sándor's hypothesis concerning reticular formation mediation in the large-scale neural response activated during Calatonia has been borne out by subsequent research based on brain imaging (fMRI-PET, EEG, NIRS). Here, we articulate an updated argument in the light of this evidence for the therapeutic benefit of engaging the orienting reflex through novel stimulation and the cognitive re-evaluation this may engender.

The functional circuitry of the reticular formation (RF), known as the reticular activating system (RAS), has long been recognized as a central component within a multitude of subcortical and cortical neural circuitry [81]. The RAS has been implicated in cognitive functions such as the orienting reflex to novel stimuli [7], attention, sleep, homeostatic regulation, as well as the transmission and modulation of pain, alongside other brain structures [82–85]. Essentially, the RF plays a major role in the modulation of attention to the extremely light sensory stimuli of Calatonia, which takes the organism by surprise and induces an orienting reflex, with extensive engagement of the RF and related networks in this process.

The OR triggers an extensive search for possible associations to previous contexts and meanings within the individual's history, beginning with short-term memories and moving on to those that may be embedded in implicit memory. With the aim of associating the new stimulus to previous memory representations, the brain quickly 'explores' the memory via the hippocampus and sensory association areas in the central-parietal cortex. In this process, a set of neocortical limbic interactions occur to resolve the significance of the stimulus [73,86,87].

Uddin and colleagues [88] note that the insula is commonly involved in detection of novel stimuli across sensory modalities. The insula, dorsal anterior cingulate (dACC) and other subcortical structures form part of the 'salience network' (SN), which is activated in response to out-of-the-ordinary or "oddball" stimuli. The function of the SN is to identify "the most homeostatically relevant among multiple competing internal and external stimuli" [88]. Most importantly, for the higher-order cognitive processes produced with Calatonia [17] where more complex stimuli require greater cognitive processing, the dorsal anterior insula will be recruited. Insular activation primarily functions "to integrate external sensory information with internal emotional and bodily state signals to coordinate brain network dynamics and to initiate switches between the default mode network (DMN) and central executive network (CEN)" [88].

If no associations are formed between the tactile stimuli in Calatonia and previous experiences recorded as memories, then the significance of the event will be assessed primarily by the amygdala. The amygdala plays an important role in encoding, storing and retrieving emotionally charged events and controlling the hormonal cascade triggered by defensive responses [89]. Amygdalar structures are activated by both emotionally salient and novel stimuli. This activation may occur regardless of whether the stimuli are emotionally valent and/or pleasant or unpleasant. In addition, the salience of the emotion is central to determining whether either a fight-or-flight or other motivational or appetitive response is triggered [90–94].

8. The Appraisal of New Stimuli

A stimulus or event is significant if it is helpful in satisfying a need, reaching a goal, or sustaining an internal value. The opposite holds true for negative significance, whereupon the stimulus is unhelpful for achieving any of the aforementioned goals. In ANS terminology, significance can be equated to homeostasis, whereby a stimulus or event positively influences homeostatic mechanisms, leading to that stimulus being attributed a high level of significance [92,95,96].

Scherer [97] asserts that the appraisal of significance is defined by one's needs, goals, values and general wellbeing, which leads to a cascade of motivation-related changes. In particular, emotionally-laden appraisals of pleasantness and well-being (or the opposite valence) lead to somatovisceral changes via the ANS and changes in motor facial expression, as well as voice and bodily tensions, conveyed through the somatic nervous system [97–99]. Over the course of Calatonia, adjustments in body tension are frequently reported in the form of twitching, sudden jerks, spontaneous jolts felt in the diaphragm, lung expansion (a respiratory reflex) and fluttering eyelids, while at the end of Calatonia, the facial muscles are often notably relaxed [17–20,32].

In the presence of a pleasant OR, several somatic responses may occur, such as a deceleration in heart rate, salivation, pupillary responses, pharyngeal expansion and a relaxation of the tract walls ('wide voice') [97]. These many somatic reactions are conducive to a trophotropic response (a relaxation response for resting and replenishing energy) and increased stability. This may in turn lead to a decrease in respiration rate, a slight decrease in heart rate, sphincter relaxation, a decrease in general muscle tone, relaxation in facial muscle tone and overall relaxation of the vocal apparatus ('relaxed voice'), comfort and resting posture. If this relaxation response leads to changes in one's motivational state and plans for action, an ergotropic shift (the activation response and usage of energy) may occur as a result of experiencing well-being [97]—in this way, one feels motivated to become proactive. This fact may explain why Calatonia is a method of psychophysiological regulation and not exclusively a relaxation technique because, ultimately, it takes the organism where it needs to go. Whether positively activated (ergotropic) or relaxed (trophotropic), Calatonia fosters the organism's optimal state [17–20].

9. ORs in Clinical Practice

The emotional significance of a stimulus, defined by its level of pleasantness and importance, can frequently affect OR intensity when focusing one's attention on a stimulus [7,100,101]. One example of the use of OR in clinical practice is a simple technique designed by Sándor: a sequence of three slow and sustained 'insufflation (blowing) on and above the seventh cervical vertebra (C4–C7)'. The therapist applies the technique while the patient remains in a sitting or standing position. This somatosensory contact at C4–C7 affects the entirety of the brachial plexus, which innervates the arm muscles, thus affecting a large area of the brain, as well as cervical vagus branching [102], causing an immediate and involuntary shift in attention with a pleasant affective tone. This is an effective way of peacefully redirecting disruptive behavior in children in less than a couple of minutes and one that has been applied on many previous occasions to institutionalized children in foster care when they felt themselves unable to engage in emotional regulation [17]. For these children, the novelty of tactile stimulation diverted their attention from an overwhelming state of emotional reaction, offering them a state of adaptive relief directly proportional to this initial state.

The process of neocortical-limbic connectivity and integration linked to an OR is not a standard occurrence in children and adults with histories of abuse and/or PTSD [103–105]. These patients frequently show symptoms of excessive limbic system activity (particularly an abnormally overactive amygdala) with less activity in the neocortex, which causes them to react impulsively to the minor triggers of daily life [106]. However, in several cases of PTSD, the opposite pattern of activation is observed, with over-activation of the prefrontal systems and over-inhibition of the amygdala and insula, leading these patients to experience flat affective states and anhedonia.

When the amygdala is chronically activated in response to trauma, stress and/or overwhelming fear, the individual's emotional response to sensory inputs becomes compromised and often requires re-setting [68,69,83]. The effects of exposure to traumatic events on brain structure and function are extensive and very specific brain regions have been implicated in trauma and PTSD [107–111]. Significant research has been dedicated towards investigating a variety of psychological treatments to address specific types of such neural dysregulation [3,112–117].

In the treatment of trauma, by prompting a neutral/pleasant OR, Calatonia shifts the patient's experience away from defensive states, leading to the re-setting of vigilant states and attentional processes and facilitating the reinstatement of neocortical–limbic interactions.

By enhancing the perception of a stimulus, Calatonia also activates motivational (or appetitive) systems that support survival, adaptation and tending to one's needs and, consequently, attentional processes based on 'interest', 'curiosity' and 'well-being'. This seemingly simple process conceals a complex reorganization of the individual on physical, emotional and cognitive levels—a process of great psychotherapeutic utility [28–30,32–34,112].

In terms of its general application in psychotherapy, the OR has been hypothesized as one of the key drivers for successful clinical outcomes following eye movement desensitization and reprocessing (EMDR) [117]. This technique aims to gradually expose the patient to the stimuli underlying PTSD and other trauma disorders, similar to other forms of cognitive-behavioral therapy. Hypothetically, EMDR pairs the recall of a traumatic event with a supposedly emotionally-neutral motor stimulus—eye movements. EMDR appears to show similar improvements in post-therapy outcomes to other cognitive-behavioral therapies particularly for the treatment of PTSD, however the functional mechanisms underlying its action remain unclear [117–120].

To many patients who suffer from PTSD, the idea of re-experiencing the trauma as proposed in EMDR is unbearable. Unlike EMDR, Calatonia does not target a specific event or memory. Consequently, there is no resetting of new homeostatic values based on previous traumatic experiences, thus amplifying the effects of Calatonia beyond specific trauma memories. Instead, there is a decrease in startle and defensive reflexes and a reinforcing of the "benign present", allowing the individual to be spontaneously released into a 'stream of consciousness' state corresponding to the emergence of the default mode network (DMN) of broad frontoparietal activation in the brain [17]. In this context, high-priority psychological issues may emerge spontaneously and rescript themselves in light of this new experience, producing the myriad of idiosyncratic reports that demonstrate the nonlinearity of psychological processes, followed by a sense of well-being [30].

10. Habituation: Does Repeated Calatonia Cease to Generate an OR?

What happens when Calatonia is repeated on a weekly basis? Does it lose its novel impact and stop triggering an OR response?

First, a description of the technique and the consent given by the patient are always requirements to minimize the possibility of a startle or defensive response by making the technique 'cognitively safe' and, evidently, this technique is offered only once a good therapeutic relationship is formed. However, a description of this technique does not prevent an OR from occurring as the OR is a result of the direct tactile stimulus and frequently resistant to top-down modulation.

In time, the sequence of touches becomes predictable and thus provides a sense of safety to the patient. Most importantly, what happens within one's mind, body and emotions during each Calatonia session may become an element of significance for an OR. The route taken towards eliciting an OR may be the same, but the journey is always different. This approach places emphasis on the significance of the event and its capacity to continue to generate a significant OR response. It is very common for patients who receive regular Calatonia to say, "today was different, I didn't feel the same way I felt last week", "today the touch seemed much lighter", "the left side of my body seemed to be heavier", or similar such observations. These comparisons can be accounted for by Friston's free energy principle [121], in which the brain is constantly trying to predict events to minimize errors. In this hypothesis, bottom-up processes are thought to compare previous events (memories) to current perceptual inputs to estimate the error in deviation between the internal model and novel input, thus recognizing minimal differences in deviation. Any changes in the representation or original "neural model" of an event that triggered an OR will retrigger the OR by establishing a comparison to what was previously experienced [122,123].

11. A Clinical Vignette

The reorganization of the (appetitive) motivational system prompted by Calatonia can be seen in action in a clinical case presenting a dysfunction of the primary motivational behavior for survival, eating. For three consecutive sessions, a fifteen-year-old female patient suffering from anorexia nervosa reported that she "knew exactly what she was going to eat for dinner". She proceeded to describe to the therapist the meal that came to her mind during the session of Calatonia.

She spontaneously sent pictures of her meals to the therapist shortly following these sessions. These included pictures of her breakfast on the mornings following therapy, revealing nutritious and complete meals. It can be hypothesized that the neurobiological mechanisms set in motion by ORs bypassed her voluntary resistance to homeostatic self-regulation and allostatic behaviors [17], restoring a biological imperative, via "neural circuits in the mammalian brain that prompt specific somatic and autonomic responses associated with motivated behavior" [9].

As the sessions of Calatonia progressed, the sadness and depression she felt surrounding her self-destructive behavior emerged—and her menstrual periods returned, along with these emotions.

In her ninth session, she reported a dream in which she "had been kidnapped by a skinny and weak man, from whom she escaped to a shopping mall together with a beautiful girl of the same age who was also his hostage".

The attentional and motivational processes set in motion during Calatonia seemed to have redirected her perception of her physical needs, revealing the pain she inflicted on herself. In the dream, the self-destructive dynamics that required her awareness were depicted by the skinny and weak man (anorexic thought patterns) and the beautiful girl (her idealized version of herself). She also began to go out more often instead of staying at home watching videos of other anorexic girls. This process suggests what Schomaker and Meeter [124] describe as an "attentional response to novelty, possibly mediated by the amygdala, an arousal-like response to deviance, which could be mediated by the noradrenergic system and a slower upregulation of exploration, motivation and learning, mediated by the dopaminergic system", as well as a possible reorganization of thalamic functional connectivity [125,126].

12. Conclusions

Calatonia and other ST techniques appear to function through the re-calibration of a subset of attentional processes. These include a reduction in the startle response to anxiety- and fear-inducing stimuli and may help to orient the patient towards novel unknown stimuli in a context of adaptation. The redirection of alerting and defensive responses towards motivational and appetitive states through innocuous, pleasant and unusual touch sequences allows the patient to implicitly process past states of trauma. A necessary prerequisite for this technique to be considered a safe psychotherapeutic approach is for the psychotherapist to have adequate training and observe strict adherence to the established protocol of touch and engagement with the patient.

Many studies discuss whether the novelty or significance of an event is the actual trigger of an OR and the consensus is that both novelty and significance are involved in the generation of an orienting response. However, significance was found to be a key factor in sustaining engagement in an OR [7,127], only a relevant/significant novel stimulus will continue to trigger an OR.

In summary, novelty-driven stimulation can support reward processes, drive exploration and other adaptive cognitive processes and enhance perception and sharpen its responses. Most importantly, an OR has a lasting and strong impact on memory and on the attentional system mediated by the amygdala, resulting from neural plasticity and deep changes to the motivational system [124].

13. Final Considerations

Beyond the impact of orienting reflexes, there are several other neurobiological, neuro-cognitive and neuro affective-emotional elements that influence the results and responses to the complex stimuli proposed in Calatonia, as listed in a previous publication [30] and briefly mentioned below.

Among these elements, dyadic regulation proposes a fine-tuned, non-verbal, inter-brain synchronization, whereby inter-brain synchronization between two individuals is defined as a natural occurrence that impacts interpersonal communication [128–132].

The importance of establishing a conscious pace of communication in therapeutic relationships cannot be emphasized enough [133–135] as several physiological systems follow a preset tempo or rhythm (heartbeat, respiration, thalamo-cortical oscillations) and "rhythms are a prominent signature of brain activity" [136]. The modulation of cortical oscillation via paced somatosensory stimuli may also facilitate integration of the individual's basic notion of selfhood. From early infancy to adulthood, selfhood is built through physical contact and proximal interaction with others via skin-to-skin interactions—before one develops the ability to share mental states in distal face-to-face interactions [137–140].

Other hypotheses about the possible elements involved in the complex mental stimuli and contexts observed in Calatonia include:

The use of (task-free) resting-state functional connectivity to facilitate access to spontaneous and pertinent (to psychotherapy) self-reflective cognitive processes [141,142];

(a) The modulation of global brain connectivity and patterns of synchronization (identified as an aspect of brain self-regulation) through the rhythmic segregation and integration of neural populations acting in concert to code for complex stimuli [143–149];
(b) The engagement of cross-hemispheric communication via the corpus callosum, which facilitates integrative higher-order neural network processes and is implicated in the ability to verbally identify, interpret and communicate emotions [150–154].
(c) The simultaneous engagement of low threshold (sensitive to light touch) skin receptors from the affective-affiliative system in the mammalian nervous system, primarily composed of C-tactile fibers and/or receptors [155–159], polymodal C-receptors, unmyelinated free nerve endings [160] and the low threshold discriminative-spatial system, associated with Merkel's cell–neurite complex receptors and Ruffini corpuscle proprioceptors [47,137,161–165].
(d) The combination of attentional systems engaged in processing the location and quality of touch, particularly the midline fronto-parietal system activated by the task-positive network, an associative network with extensive bilateral connections with other areas of the brain [127,144,166];

In conclusion, there is significant support for the importance of integrating the orienting reflex in psychotherapy through both physical and non-physical cues. ORs appear to play a mediating role in the improved behavioral outcomes from Calatonia, by initially restoring psychophysical regulation and well-being—and eventually leading to a more positive sense of self. In patients with a history of trauma or attachment issues, this may mean establishing a context of safety within individual boundaries first, through dyadic regulation, before addressing psychological issues that may lead to more feelings of vulnerability [1,167].

Author Contributions: Conceptualization, A.R.B.; writing—original draft preparation, A.R.B.; writing—review and editing, W.E.C.; visualization, A.R.B and W.E.C.; supervision, W.E.C.; project administration, A.R.B. and W.E.C.; funding acquisition, N/A. All authors have read and agreed to the published version of the manuscript.

Funding: This research received no external funding.

Conflicts of Interest: The authors declare no conflict of interest.

References

1. Fiskum, C. Psychotherapy Beyond All the Words: Dyadic Expansion, Vagal Regulation, and Biofeedback in Psychotherapy. *J. Psychother. Integr.* **2019**, *29*, 412–425. [CrossRef]
2. Knaster, M. *Discovering the Body's Wisdom: A Comprehensive Guide to more than Fifty Mind-Body Practices That Can Relieve Pain, Reduce Stress, and Foster Health, Spiritual Growth, and Inner Peace*; Bantam: New York, NY, USA, 1996.
3. Van der Kolk, B. *The Body Keeps the Score: Brain, Mind, and Body in the Healing of Trauma*; Penguin Books: New York, NY, USA, 2015.
4. Field, T. *Complementary and Alternative Therapies Research*; American Psychological Association: Washington, DC, USA, 2009.
5. Anderson, J.G.; Taylor, A.G. Effects of Healing Touch in Clinical Practice: A Systematic Review of Randomized Clinical Trials. *J. Holist. Nurs.* **2011**, *29*, 221–228. [CrossRef] [PubMed]
6. Tantia, J.F. Toward a Somatically-Informed Paradigm in Embodied Research. *Int. Body Psychother. J.* **2019**, *18*, 134–145.
7. Bradley, M.M. Natural selective attention: Orienting and emotion. *Psychophysiology* **2009**, *46*, 1–11. [CrossRef] [PubMed]
8. Miller, W. Motivational Interviewing: III. On the Ethics of Motivational Intervention. *Behav. Cogn. Psychother.* **1994**, *22*, 111–123. [CrossRef]
9. Bradley, M.M.; Codispoti, M.; Cuthbert, B.N.; Lang, P. Emotion and Motivation I: Defensive and Appetitive Reactions in Picture Processing. *Emotion* **2001**, *1*, 276–298. [CrossRef]

10. Harmon-Jones, E.; Harmon-Jones, C.; Summerell, E. On the Importance of Both Dimensional and Discrete Models of Emotion. *Behav. Sci.* **2017**, *7*, 66. [CrossRef]
11. Panksepp, J. Neurologizing the psychology of affects: How appraisal-based constructivism and basic emotion theory can coexist. *Perspect. Psychol. Sci.* **2007**, *2*, 281–296. [CrossRef]
12. Weiqi, Z.; Ye, L.; Hong, L.C.; Yu-Hsin, C.; Qian, C.; Xiaolan, F. The Influence of Event Valence and Emotional States on the Metaphorical Comprehension of Time. *Front. Psychol.* **2019**, *10*, 410.
13. Lang, P.J. Emotion and Motivation: Toward Consensus Definitions and a Common Research Purpose. *Emot. Rev.* **2010**, *2*, 229–233. [CrossRef]
14. Vrtička, P.; Vuilleumier, P. Neuroscience of human social interactions and adult attachment style. *Front. Hum. Neurosci.* **2012**, *6*, 212. [CrossRef] [PubMed]
15. Barrós-Loscertales, A.; Ventura-Campos, N.; Sanjuán-Tomás, A.; Belloch, V.; Parcet, M.A.; Avila, C. Behavioral activation system modulation on brain activation during appetitive and aversive stimulus processing. *Soc. Cogn. Affect. Neurosci.* **2010**, *5*, 18–28. [CrossRef] [PubMed]
16. Grossman, S.P. Motivation, Aversive, Biological Bases. In *States of Brain and Mind. Readings from the Encyclopedia of Neuroscience Series*; Hobson, J.A., Ed.; Birkhäuser: Boston, MA, USA, 1988; pp. 63–65.
17. Blanchard, A.R. Calatonia: Novel Insights from Neuroscience. In *Calatonia: A Therapeutic Approach that Promotes Somatic and Psychological Regulation*; Blanchard, A.R., Rios, A.M.G., Seixas, L.P., Eds.; Alma Street Enterprise: Miami, FL, USA, 2019; pp. 286–304.
18. Farah, R. *Calatonia: Subtle Touch in Psychotherapy*; Companhia Ilimitada: São Paulo, Brazil, 2017.
19. Sándor, P. Calatonia. *Bol. De Psicol.* **1969**, *XXI*, 92–100.
20. Sándor, P. Calatonia. In *Calatonia: A Therapeutic Approach that Promotes Somatic and Psychological Regulation*; Blanchard, A.R., Rios, A.M.G., Seixas, L.P., Eds.; Alma Street Enterprise: Miami, FL, USA, 2019; pp. 1–13.
21. Armando, M.D. Calatonia and Resillience. In *Calatonia: A Therapeutic Approach that Promotes Somatic and Psychological Regulation*; Blanchard, A.R., Rios, A.M.G., Seixas, L.P., Eds.; Alma Street Enterprise: Miami, FL, USA, 2019; pp. 263–285.
22. Insel, T.; Cuthbert, B.; Garvey, M.; Heinssen, R.; Pine, D.S.; Quinn, K.; Sanislow, C.; Wang, P. Research domain criteria (RDoC): Toward a new classification framework for research on mental disorders. *Am. J. Psychiatry* **2010**, *167*, 167–748. [CrossRef]
23. Gupta, A.; Love, A.; Kilpatrick, L.A.; Labus, J.S.; Bhatt, R.; Chang, L.; Tillisch, K.; Naliboff, B.; Mayer, E.A. Morphological Brain Measures of Cortico-Limbic Inhibition Related to Resilience. *J. Neurosci. Res.* **2017**, *95*, 1760–1775. [CrossRef]
24. Farah, R. The Academic Teaching of Calatonia. In *Calatonia: A Therapeutic Approach that Promotes Somatic and Psychological Regulation*; Blanchard, A.R., Rios, A.M.G., Seixas, L.P., Eds.; Alma Street Enterprise: Miami, FL, USA, 2019; pp. 26–45.
25. Machado Filho, P.T. The Legacy of Sándor. In *Calatonia: A Therapeutic Approach that Promotes Somatic and Psychological Regulation*; Blanchard, A.R., Rios, A.M.G., Seixas, L.P., Eds.; Alma Street Enterprise: Miami, FL, USA, 2019; pp. 14–25.
26. Kirsch, T. *The Jungians*; Routledge: London, UK, 2000.
27. Delmanto, S. *Subtle Touches: Calatonia, A Life Experience with Pethö Sándor's Work*; Summus: São Paulo, Brazil, 2008.
28. Gonçalves, M.I.C.; Pereira, M.A.; Ribeiro, A.J.; Rios, A.M.G. Subtle touch, calatonia and other somatic interventions with children and adolescents. *Int. Body Psychother. J.* **2007**, *6*, 33–47.
29. Rios, A.M.G.; Seixas, L.P.; Blanchard, A.R. The Body in Psychotherapy: Calatonia and Subtle Touch Techniques. In *Body, Mind, and Healing After Jung: A Space of Questions*; Jones, R., Ed.; Routledge: London, UK, 2010; pp. 228–250.
30. Blanchard, A.R.; Rios, A.M.G.; Seixas, L.P. (Eds.) *Calatonia: A Therapeutic Approach that Promotes Somatic and Psychological Regulation*; Alma Street Enterprise: Miami, FL, USA, 2019.
31. Morrison, I. Keep Calm and Cuddle on: Social Touch as a Stress Buffer. *Adapt. Hum. Behav. Physiol.* **2016**, *2*, 344–362. [CrossRef]
32. Greger Tavares, S.M.; Vannuchi, B.P.; Machado, F.P.T.; Andrade, A.L.M. Efeitos psicofisiológicos da Calatonia em adultos: Um estudo piloto na abordagem quanti-qualitativa. *Jung Corpo* **2015**, *15*, 17–33.

33. Lasaponari, E.F. A Utilização Da Calatonia No Período Pós-Operatório Imediato. Unpublished. Master's Thesis, Nursing School, University of São Paulo, São Paulo, Brazil, 2011. Available online: http://www.teses.usp.br/teses/disponiveis/7/7139/tde-21062011-152045/ (accessed on 6 February 2020).
34. Nossow, V.; Peniche, A.C.G. Paciente cirurgico ambulatorial: Calatonia e ansiedade. *Acta Paul. De Enferm.* **2007**, *20*, 161–167. [CrossRef]
35. Löken, L.S.; Olausson, H. The skin as a social organ. *Exp. Brain Res.* **2010**, *204*, 305–314.
36. Craig, A.D. How do you feel? Interoception: The sense of the physiological condition of the body. *Nat. Rev. Neurosci.* **2002**, *3*, 655–666. [CrossRef] [PubMed]
37. Craig, A.D. Interoception and emotion: A neuroanatomical perspective. In *Handbook of Emotions*; Lewis, M., Haviland-Jones, J.M., Feldman Barrett, L., Eds.; The Guildford Press: New York, NY, USA, 2008; pp. 272–288.
38. Löken, L.S.; Wessberg, J.; Morrison, I.; McGlone, F.; Olausson, H. Coding of pleasant touch by unmyelinated afferents in humans. *Nat. Neurosci.* **2009**, *12*, 547–548. [CrossRef] [PubMed]
39. Moehring, F.; Halder, P.; Seal, R.P.; Stucky, C.L. Uncovering the cells and circuits of touch in normal and pathological settings. *Neuron* **2018**, *100*, 349–360. [CrossRef] [PubMed]
40. Abraham, J.; Mathew, S. Merkel Cells: A Collective Review of Current Concepts. *Int. J. Appl. Basic Med. Res.* **2019**, *9*, 9–13.
41. Chang, W.; Kanda, H.; Ikeda, R.; Ling, J.; DeBerry, J.J.; Gu, J.G. Merkel disc is a serotonergic synapse in the epidermis for transmitting tactile signals in mammals. *Proc. Natl. Acad. Sci. USA* **2016**, *113*, E5491–E5500. [CrossRef] [PubMed]
42. Halata, Z.; Grim, M.; Baumann, K.I. Current understanding of Merkel cells, touch reception and the skin. *Expert Rev. Dermatol.* **2010**, *5*, 109–116. [CrossRef]
43. Johansson, R.S.; Vallbo, A.B. Tactile sensibility in the human hand: Relative and absolute densities of four types of mechanoreceptive units in glabrous skin. *J. Physiol.* **1979**, *286*, 283–300. [CrossRef]
44. Johansson, R.S.; Vallbo, Å.B. Tactile sensory coding in the glabrous skin of the human hand. *Trends Neurosci.* **1983**, *6*, 27–32. [CrossRef]
45. Maksimovic, S.; Baba, Y.; Lumpkin, E.A. Neurotransmitters and synaptic components in the Merkel cell-neurite complex, a gentle touch receptor. *Ann. N. Y. Acad. Sci.* **2013**, *1279*, 13–21. [CrossRef]
46. Maksimovic, S.; Nakatani, M.; Baba, Y.; Nelson, A.M.; Marshall, K.L.; Wellnitz, S.A.; Firozi, P.; Woo, S.H.; Ranade, S.; Patapoutian, A.; et al. Epidermal Merkel cells are mechanosensory cells that tune mammalian touch receptors. *Nature* **2014**, *509*, 617–621. [CrossRef]
47. McGlone, F.; Wessberg, J.; Olausson, H. Discriminative and Affective Touch: Sensing and Feeling. *Neuron* **2014**, *82*, 737–755. [CrossRef] [PubMed]
48. Rolls, E.T. The affective and cognitive processing of touch, oral texture, and temperature in the brain. *Neurosci. Biobehav. Rev.* **2010**, *34*, 237–245. [CrossRef] [PubMed]
49. Hayward, V. A Brief Overview of the Human Somatosensory System. In *Musical Haptics*; Papetti, S., Saitis, C., Eds.; Springer: Cham, Switzerland, 2018; pp. 29–48.
50. Millar, S. *Reading by Touch*; Routledge: New York, NY, USA, 1997.
51. Klooster, N.B.; Cook, S.W.; Uc, E.Y.; Duff, M.C. Gestures make memories, but what kind? Patients with impaired procedural memory display disruptions in gesture production and comprehension. *Front. Hum. Neurosci.* **2015**, *8*, 1054. [CrossRef] [PubMed]
52. Squire, L.R.; Dede, A.J. Conscious and unconscious memory systems. *Cold Spring Harb. Perspect. Biol.* **2015**, *7*, a021667. [CrossRef]
53. Allum, J.H.J.; Bloem, B.R.; Carpenter, M.G.; Hulliger, M.; Hadders-Algra, M. Proprioceptive control of posture: A review of new concepts. *Gait Posture* **1998**, *8*, 214–242. [CrossRef]
54. Drew, T.; Prentice, S.; Schepens, B. Cortical and brainstem control of locomotion. *Prog. Brain Res.* **2004**, *143*, 251–261.
55. Kennedy, P.M.; Inglis, J.T. Distribution and behaviour of glabrous cutaneous receptors in the human foot sole. *J. Physiol.* **2002**, *538*, 995–1002. [CrossRef]
56. Malcuit, G.; Bastien, C.; Pomerleau, A. Habituation of the orienting response to stimuli of different functional values in 4-month-old infants. *J. Exp. Child Psychol.* **1996**, *62*, 272–291. [CrossRef]
57. Buodo, G.; Sarlo, M.; Palomba, D. Attentional resources measured by reaction times highlight differences within pleasant and unpleasant, high arousing stimuli. *Motiv. Emot.* **2002**, *26*, 123–138. [CrossRef]

58. Fan, J.; McCandliss, B.D.; Fossella, J.; Flombaum, J.I.; Posner, M. The activation of attentional networks. *NeuroImage* **2005**, *26*, 471–479. [CrossRef]
59. Lang, P.J.; Bradley, M.M. Appetitive and Defensive Motivation: Goal-Directed or Goal-Determined? *Emot. Rev. J. Int. Soc. Res. Emot.* **2013**, *5*, 230–234. [CrossRef] [PubMed]
60. Posner, M.I.; Petersen, S.E. The Attention System of the Human Brain. *Annu. Rev. Neurosci.* **2003**, *13*, 25–42. [CrossRef] [PubMed]
61. Ross-Sheehy, S.; Schneegans, S.; Spencer, J.P. The Infant Orienting with Attention task: Assessing the neural basis of spatial attention in infancy. *Infancy Off. J. Int. Soc. Infant Stud.* **2015**, *20*, 467–506. [CrossRef] [PubMed]
62. Williams, L.M.; Brammer, M.J.; Skerrett, D.; Lagopolous, J.; Rennie, C.; Kozek, K.; Olivieri, G.; Peduto, T.; Gordon, E. The neural correlates of orienting: An integration of fMRI and skin conductance orienting. *Neuroreport* **2000**, *11*, 3011–3015. [CrossRef] [PubMed]
63. Geva, R.; Zivan, M.; Warsha, A.; Olchik, D. Alerting, orienting or executive attention networks: Differential patterns of pupil dilations. *Front. Behav. Neurosci.* **2013**, *7*, 145. [CrossRef]
64. Posner, M.I. *Attention in the Social World*; Oxford University Press: New York, NY, USA, 2012.
65. Posner, M.I. Attentional networks and consciousness. *Front. Psychol.* **2012**, *3*, 64. [CrossRef]
66. Pavlov, I.P. *Conditioned Reflexes*; Oxford University Press: Oxford, UK, 1927.
67. Loewenstein, G. The psychology of curiosity: A review and reinterpretation. *Psychol. Bull.* **1994**, *116*, 75–98. [CrossRef]
68. DeGangi, G.A. *The Dysregulated Adult: Integrated Treatment Approaches*; Academic Press: Cambridge, MA, USA, 2012.
69. DeGangi, G.A. *Pediatric Disorders of Regulation in Affect and Behavior: A Therapist's Guide to Assessment and Treatment*; Academic Press: Cambridge, MA, USA, 2017.
70. Sokolov, E.N. *Perception and the Conditioned Reflex*; Macmillan: New York, NY, USA, 1963.
71. Bradley, M.M.; Keil, A.; Lang, P.J. Orienting and Emotional Perception: Facilitation, Attenuation, and Interference. *Front. Psychol.* **2012**, *3*, 493. [CrossRef]
72. Graham, F.K.; Clifton, R.K. Heart-rate change as a component of the orienting response. *Psychol. Bull.* **1966**, *65*, 305–320. [CrossRef]
73. Bernstein, A.S. The Orienting Response as Novelty and Significance Detector: Reply to O'Gorman. *Psychophysiology* **1979**, *16*, 263–273. [CrossRef]
74. Sambo, C.F.; Forster, B. Sustained Spatial Attention in Touch: Modality-Specific and Multimodal Mechanisms. *Sci. World J.* **2011**, *11*, 199–213. [CrossRef] [PubMed]
75. Engbert, K.; Wohlschläger, A.; Haggard, P. Who is causing what? The sense of agency is relational and efferent-triggered. *Cognition* **2008**, *107*, 693–704. [CrossRef] [PubMed]
76. Mangalam, M.; Cutts, S.A.; Fragaszy, D.M. Sense of ownership and not the sense of agency is spatially bounded within the space reachable with the unaugmented hand. *Exp. Brain Res.* **2019**, *237*, 2911–2924. [CrossRef] [PubMed]
77. Tsakiris, M.; Schütz-Bosbach, S.; Gallagher, S. On agency and body-ownership: Phenomenological and neurocognitive reflections. *Conscious. Cogn.* **2007**, *16*, 645–660. [CrossRef]
78. Tomkins, S. *Affect Imagery Consciousness, Vol I: The Positive Affects*; Springer: New York, NY, USA, 1962.
79. Stevens, C.; Bavelier, D. The role of selective attention on academic foundations: A cognitive neuroscience perspective. *Dev. Cogn. Neurosci.* **2012**, *2*, S30–S48. [CrossRef] [PubMed]
80. Harjunen, V.J.; Spapé, M.; Ahmed, I.; Jacucci, G.; Ravaja, N. Individual differences in affective touch: Behavioral inhibition and gender define how an interpersonal touch is perceived. *Personal. Individ. Differ.* **2017**, *107*, 88–95. [CrossRef]
81. Parvizi, J.; Damasio, A. Consciousness and the brain-stem. *Cognition* **2001**, *79*, 135–160. [CrossRef]
82. Martins, I.; Tavares, I. Reticular Formation and Pain: The Past and the Future. *Front. Neuroanat.* **2017**, *11*, 51. [CrossRef]
83. Neugebauer, V. Chapter 15: Amygdala pain mechanisms. In *Handbook of Experimental Pharmacology*; Barrett, J.E., Ed.; Springer: New York, NY, USA, 2015; pp. 261–284.
84. Venkatraman, A.; Edlow, B.L.; Immordino-Yang, M.H. The Brainstem in Emotion: A Review. *Front. Neuroanat.* **2017**, *11*, 15. [CrossRef]

85. Youssef, A.M.; Macefield, V.G.; Henderson, L.A. Cortical influences on brainstem circuitry responsible for conditioned pain modulation in humans. *Hum. Brain Mapp.* **2016**, *37*, 2630–2644. [CrossRef]
86. Bremner, J.D. Traumatic stress: Effects on the brain. *Dialogues Clin. Neurosci.* **2006**, *8*, 445–461. [PubMed]
87. Jeewajee, A.; Lever, C.; Burton, S.; O'Keefe, J.; Burgess, N. Environmental novelty is signaled by reduction of the hippocampal theta frequency. *Hippocampus* **2008**, *18*, 340–348. [CrossRef] [PubMed]
88. Uddin, L.Q.; Nomi, J.S.; Hébert-Seropian, B.; Ghaziri, J.; Boucher, O. Structure and Function of the Human Insula. *J. Clin. Neurophysiol.* **2017**, *34*, 300–306. [CrossRef] [PubMed]
89. Howe, M.L.; Cicchetti, D.; Toth, S.L. Children's basic memory processes, stress, and maltreatment. *Dev. Psychopathol.* **2006**, *18*, 759–769. [CrossRef]
90. Balderston, N.L.; Schultz, D.H.; Helmstetter, F.J. The human amygdala plays a stimulus specific role in the detection of novelty. *NeuroImage* **2011**, *55*, 1889–1898. [CrossRef] [PubMed]
91. Bonnet, L.; Comte, A.; Tatu, L.; Millot, J.-L.; Moulin, T.; Medeiros de Bustos, E. The role of the amygdala in the perception of positive emotions: An "intensity detector". *Front. Behav. Neurosci.* **2015**, *9*, 178. [CrossRef]
92. Morrison, S.E.; Salzman, C.D. Revaluing the amygdala. *Curr. Opin. Neurobiol.* **2010**, *20*, 221–230. [CrossRef]
93. Murray, E.A. The amygdala, reward and emotion. *Trends Cogn. Sci.* **2007**, *11*, 489–497. [CrossRef]
94. Weymar, M.; Schwabe, L. Amygdala and Emotion: The Bright Side of It. *Front. Neurosci.* **2016**, *10*, 224. [CrossRef]
95. Phelps, E.A.; LeDoux, J.E. Contributions of the amygdala to emotion processing: From animal models to human behavior. *Neuron* **2005**, *48*, 175–187. [CrossRef]
96. Vasa, R.A.; Pine, D.S.; Thorn, J.M.; Nelson, T.E.; Spinelli, S.; Nelson, E.; Maheu, F.S.; Ernst, M.; Bruck, M.; Mostofsky, S.H. Enhanced Right Amygdala Activity in Adolescents during Encoding of Positively-Valenced Pictures. *Dev. Cogn. Neurosci.* **2011**, *1*, 88–99. [CrossRef] [PubMed]
97. Scherer, K.R. Emotions are emergent processes: They require a dynamic computational architecture. *Philos. Trans. R. Soc. B Biol. Sci.* **2009**, *364*, 3459–3474. [CrossRef] [PubMed]
98. Blackford, J.U.; Buckholtz, J.W.; Avery, S.N.; Zald, D.H. A unique role for the human amygdala in novelty detection. *NeuroImage* **2010**, *50*, 1188–1193. [CrossRef] [PubMed]
99. Vuilleumier, P. How brains beware: Neural mechanisms of emotional attention. *Trends Cogn. Sci.* **2005**, *9*, 585–594. [CrossRef]
100. Lang, P.J.; Bradley, M.M. Emotion and the motivational brain. *Biol. Psychol.* **2010**, *84*, 437–450. [CrossRef]
101. Schomaker, J.; Rangel-Gomez, M.; Meeter, M. Happier, faster: Developmental changes in the effects of mood and novelty on responses. *Q. J. Exp. Psychol.* **2016**, *69*, 37–47. [CrossRef]
102. Hammer, N.; Glätzner, J.; Feja, C.; Kühne, C.; Meixensberger, J.; Planitzer, U.; Schleifenbaum, S.; Tillmann, B.N.; Winkler, D. Human vagus nerve branching in the cervical region. *PLoS ONE* **2015**, *10*, e0118006. [CrossRef]
103. Keding, T.J.; Herringa, R.J. Paradoxical Prefrontal—Amygdala Recruitment to Angry and Happy Expressions in Pediatric Posttraumatic Stress Disorder. *Neuropsychopharmacology* **2016**, *41*, 2903–2912. [CrossRef]
104. Marusak, H.A.; Martin, K.R.; Etkin, A.; Thomason, M.E. Childhood Trauma Exposure Disrupts the Automatic Regulation of Emotional Processing. *Neuropsychopharmacology* **2015**, *40*, 1250–1258. [CrossRef]
105. White, S.F.; Costanzo, M.E.; Blair, J.R.; Roy, M.J. PTSD symptom severity is associated with increased recruitment of top-down attentional control in a trauma-exposed sample. *Neuroimage Clin.* **2015**, *7*, 19–27. [CrossRef]
106. Streeck-Fischer, A.; van der Kolk, B.A. Down will come baby, cradle and all: Diagnostic and therapeutic implications of chronic trauma on child development. *Aust. N. Z. J. Psychiatry* **2000**, *34*, 903–918. [CrossRef] [PubMed]
107. Block, S.R.; King, A.P.; Sripada, R.K.; Weissman, D.H.; Welsh, R.; Liberzon, I. Behavioral and neural correlates of disrupted orienting attention in posttraumatic stress disorder. *Cogn. Affect. Behav. Neurosci.* **2017**, *17*, 422–436. [CrossRef] [PubMed]
108. Teicher, M.H.; Alaptagin, K. Childhood maltreatment, cortical and amygdala morphometry, functional connectivity, laterality, and psychopathology. *Child Maltreat.* **2019**, *24*, 458–465. [CrossRef] [PubMed]
109. Butler, O.; Adolf, J.; Gleich, T.; Willmund, G.; Zimmermann, P.; Lindenberger, U.; Gallinat, J.; Kühn, S. Military deployment correlates with smaller prefrontal gray matter volume and psychological symptoms in a subclinical population. *Transl. Psychiatry* **2017**, *7*, e1031. [CrossRef]

110. Kim, S.; Kim, J.S.; Jin, M.J.; Im, C.-H.; Lee, S.-H. Dysfunctional frontal lobe activity during inhibitory tasks in individuals with childhood trauma: An event-related potential study. *Neuroimage Clin.* **2018**, *17*, 935–942. [CrossRef]
111. Sherin, J.E.; Nemeroff, C.B. Post-traumatic stress disorder: The neurobiological impact of psychological trauma. *Dialogues Clin. Neurosci.* **2011**, *13*, 263–278.
112. Herbert, C. Calatonia and Subtle Touch in the Healing of Trauma. In *Calatonia: A Therapeutic Approach that Promotes Somatic and Psychological Regulation*; Blanchard, A.R., Rios, A.M.G., Seixas, L.P., Eds.; Alma Street Enterprise: Miami, FL, USA, 2019; pp. 70–86.
113. Herbert, C. *Overcoming Traumatic Stress—A Self-Help Guide Using Cognitive Behavioural Techniques*; Robinson, Little Brown Book Group: London, UK, 2017.
114. Resick, P.A.; Monson, C.M.; Chard, K.M. *Cognitive Processing Therapy for PTSD: A Comprehensive Manual*; Guilford Press: New York, NY, USA, 2016.
115. Ogden, P.; Minton, K.; Pain, C. *Trauma and the Body: A Sensory Motor Approach to Therapy*; W.W. Norton: New York, NY, USA, 2006.
116. Payne, P.; Levine, P.A.; Crane-Godreau, M.A. Somatic experiencing: Using interoception and proprioception as core elements of trauma therapy. *Front. Psychol.* **2015**, *6*, 93.
117. Shapiro, F.; Forrest, M.S. *EMDR: The Break-Through Therapy for Overcoming Anxiety, Stress, and Trauma*; Basic Books: New York, NY, USA, 2004.
118. Seidler, G.H.; Wagner, F.E. Comparing the efficacy of EMDR and trauma-focused cognitive-behavioral therapy in the treatment of PTSD: A meta-analytic study. *Psychol. Med.* **2006**, *36*, 1515–1522. [CrossRef]
119. Patihis, L.; Cruz, C.S.; McNally, R.J. Eye Movement Desensitization and Reprocessing (EMDR). In *Encyclopedia of Personality & Individual Differences*; Zeigler-Hill, V., Shackelford, T.K., Eds.; Springer: New York, NY, USA, 2017.
120. Chamberlin, D.E. The Predictive Processing Model of EMDR. *Front. Psychol.* **2019**, *10*, 2267. [CrossRef]
121. Friston, K. The free-energy principle: A rough guide to the brain? *Trends Cogn. Sci.* **2009**, *13*, 293–301. [CrossRef]
122. Sokolov, E.N.; Spinks, J.A.; Naatanen, R.; Lyytinen, H. *The Orienting Response in Information Processing*; Lawrence Erlbaum: Mahwah, NJ, USA, 2002.
123. Torta, D.M.; Liang, M.; Valentini, E.; Mouraux, A.; Iannetti, G.D. Dishabituation of laser-evoked EEG responses: Dissecting the effect of certain and uncertain changes in stimulus spatial location. *Exp. Brain Res.* **2012**, *218*, 361–372. [CrossRef] [PubMed]
124. Schomaker, J.; Meeter, M. Short- and long-lasting consequences of novelty, deviance and surprise on brain and cognition. *Neurosci. Biobehav. Rev.* **2015**, *55*, 268–279. [CrossRef] [PubMed]
125. Harshaw, C. Interoceptive dysfunction: Toward an integrated framework for understanding somatic and affective disturbance in depression. *Psychol. Bull.* **2015**, *141*, 311–363. [CrossRef] [PubMed]
126. Kang, L.; Zhang, A.; Sun, N.; Liu, P.; Yang, C.; Li, G.; Liu, Z.; Wang, Y.; Zhang, K. Functional connectivity between the thalamus and the primary somatosensory cortex in major depressive disorder: A resting-state fMRI study. *BMC Psychiatry* **2018**, *18*, 339. [CrossRef] [PubMed]
127. Daffner, K.R.; Scinto, L.F.; Weitzman, A.M.; Faust, R.; Rentz, D.M.; Budson, A.E.; Holcomb, P.J. Frontal and parietal components of a cerebral network mediating voluntary attention to novel events. *J. Cogn. Neurosci.* **2003**, *15*, 294–313. [CrossRef]
128. Cacioppo, S.; Zhou, H.; Monteleone, G.; Majka, E.A.; Quinn, K.A.; Ball, A.B.; Norman, G.J.; Semin, G.R.; Cacioppo, J.T. You are in sync with me: Neural correlates of interpersonal synchrony with a partner. *Neuroscience* **2014**, *277*, 842–858. [CrossRef]
129. Dumas, G.; Nadel, J.; Soussignan, R.; Martinerie, J.; Garnero, L. Inter-brain synchronization during social interaction. *PLoS ONE* **2010**, *5*, e12166. [CrossRef]
130. Hove, M.J.; Risen, J.L. It's All in the Timing: Interpersonal Synchrony Increases Affiliation. *Soc. Cogn.* **2009**, *27*, 949–960. [CrossRef]
131. Hu, Y.; Hu, Y.; Li, X.; Pan, Y.; Cheng, X. Brain-to-brain synchronization across two persons predicts mutual prosociality. *Soc. Cogn. Affect. Neurosci.* **2017**, *12*, 1835–1844. [CrossRef]
132. Mu, Y.; Guo, C.; Han, S. Oxytocin enhances inter-brain synchrony during social coordination in male adults. *Soc. Cogn. Affect. Neurosci.* **2016**, *11*, 1882–1893. [CrossRef]

133. Koole, S.L.; Tschacher, W. Synchrony in Psychotherapy: A Review and an Integrative Framework for the Therapeutic Alliance. *Front. Psychol.* **2016**, *7*, 862. [CrossRef] [PubMed]
134. Schore, A.N. Relational trauma and the developing right brain: An interface of psychoanalytic self-psychology and neuroscience. *Ann. N. Y. Acad. Sci.* **2009**, *1159*, 189–203. [CrossRef] [PubMed]
135. Siegel, D.J. *The Developing Mind*; The Guilford Press: New York, NY, USA, 2012.
136. Jones, S.R. When brain rhythms aren't 'rhythmic': Implication for their mechanisms and meaning. *Curr. Opin. Neurobiol.* **2016**, *40*, 72–80. [CrossRef] [PubMed]
137. Ciaunica, A.; Fotopoulou, A. The touched self: Psychological and philosophical perspectives on proximal intersubjectivity and the self. In *Embodiment, Enaction, and Culture: Investigating the Constitution of the Shared World*; Durt, C., Fuchs, T., Tewes, C., Eds.; MIT Press: Cambridge, MA, USA, 2017; pp. 173–192.
138. Hallam, G.P.; Webb, T.L.; Sheeran, P.; Miles, E.; Niven, K.; Wilkinson, I.D.; Hunter, M.D.; Woodruff, P.W.; Totterdell, P.; Farrow, T.F. The neural correlates of regulating another person's emotions: An exploratory fMRI study. *Front. Hum. Neurosci.* **2014**, *8*, 376. [CrossRef] [PubMed]
139. Naruse, K.; Hirai, T. Effects of slow tempo exercise on respiration, heart rate, and mood state. *Percept. Mot. Ski.* **2000**, *91*, 729–740. [CrossRef]
140. Szirmai, I. How does the brain create rhythms? *Ideggyógy. Szle.* **2010**, *63*, 13–23.
141. Deco, G.; Kringelbach, M.L.; Jirsa, V.K.; Ritter, P. The dynamics of resting fluctuations in the brain: Metastability and its dynamical cortical core. *Sci. Rep.* **2017**, *7*, 1–14. [CrossRef]
142. Smallwood, J.; Schooler, J.W. The Science of Mind Wandering: Empirically Navigating the Stream of Consciousness. *Annu. Rev. Psychol.* **2015**, *66*, 487–518. [CrossRef]
143. Bell, P.T.; Shine, J.M. Subcortical contributions to large-scale network communication. *Neurosci. Biobehav. Rev.* **2016**, *71*, 313–322. [CrossRef]
144. Goldberg, I.I.; Harel, M.; Malach, R. When the Brain Loses Its Self: Prefrontal Inactivation during Sensorimotor Processing. *Neuron* **2006**, *50*, 329–339. [CrossRef]
145. Gollo, L.L.; Zalesky, A.; Hutchison, R.M.; van den Heuvel, M.; Breakspear, M. Dwelling quietly in the rich club: Brain network determinants of slow cortical fluctuations. *Philos. Trans. R. Soc. Lond. Ser. B Biol. Sci.* **2015**, *370*, 20140165. [CrossRef] [PubMed]
146. Hari, R.; Parkkonen, L. The brain timewise: How timing shapes and supports brain function. *Philos. Trans. R. Soc. Lond. Ser. B Biol. Sci.* **2015**, *370*, 20140170. [CrossRef] [PubMed]
147. Kaiser, R.H.; Andrews-Hanna, J.R.; Wager, T.D.; Pizzagalli, D.A. Large-Scale Network Dysfunction in Major Depressive Disorder: A Meta-analysis of Resting-State Functional Connectivity. *JAMA Psychiatry* **2015**, *72*, 603–611. [CrossRef] [PubMed]
148. Park, H.J.; Friston, K. Structural and functional brain networks: From connections to cognition. *Science* **2013**, *342*, 1238411. [CrossRef]
149. Santangelo, V. Large-Scale brain networks supporting divided attention across spatial locations and sensory modalities. *Front. Integr. Neurosci.* **2018**, *12*, 8. [CrossRef] [PubMed]
150. Compton, R.J.; Carp, J.; Chaddock, L.; Fineman, S.L.; Quandt, L.C.; Ratliff, J.B. Trouble Crossing the Bridge: Altered Interhemispheric Communication of Emotional Images in Anxiety. *Emotion* **2008**, *8*, 684–692. [CrossRef] [PubMed]
151. Compton, R.J.; Feigenson, K.; Widick, P. Take it to the bridge: An interhemispheric processing advantage for emotional faces. *Cogn. Brain Res.* **2005**, *24*, 66–72. [CrossRef] [PubMed]
152. Hearne, L.J.; Dean, R.J.; Robinson, G.A.; Richards, L.J.; Mattingley, J.B.; Cocchi, L. Increased cognitive complexity reveals abnormal brain network activity in individuals with corpus callosum dysgenesis. *Neuroimage Clin.* **2019**, *21*, 101595. [CrossRef] [PubMed]
153. Roland, J.L.; Snyder, A.Z.; Hacker, C.D.; Mitra, A.; Shimony, J.S.; Limbrick, D.D.; Raichle, M.E.; Smyth, M.D.; Leuthardt, E.C. On the role of the corpus callosum in interhemispheric functional connectivity in humans. *Proc. Natl. Acad. Sci. USA* **2017**, *114*, 13278–13283. [CrossRef]
154. Skumlien, M.; Sederevicius, D.; Fjell, A.M.; Walhovd, K.B.; Westerhausen, R. Parallel but independent reduction of emotional awareness and corpus callosum connectivity in older age. *PLoS ONE* **2018**, *13*, e0209915. [CrossRef]
155. Brauer, J.; Xiao, Y.; Poulain, T.; Friederici, A.D.; Schirmer, A. Frequency of Maternal Touch Predicts Resting Activity and Connectivity of the Developing Social Brain. *Cereb. Cortex* **2016**, *26*, 3544–3552. [CrossRef] [PubMed]

156. Iggo, A. Cutaneous mechanoreceptors with afferent C fibres. *J. Physiol.* **1960**, *152*, 337–353. [CrossRef] [PubMed]
157. Iggo, A.; Muir, A.R. The structure and function of a slowly adapting touch corpuscle in hairy skin. *J. Physiol.* **1969**, *200*, 763–796. [CrossRef] [PubMed]
158. Olausson, H.; Lamarre, Y.; Backlund, H.; Morin, C.; Wallin, B.G.; Starck, G.; Ekholm, S.; Strigo, I.; Worsley, K.; Vallbo, Å.B.; et al. Unmyelinated tactile afferents signal touch and project to insular cortex. *Nat. Neurosci.* **2002**, *5*, 900–904. [CrossRef]
159. Olausson, H.; Wessberg, J.; Morrison, I.; McGlone, F.; Vallbo, Å. The neurophysiology of unmyelinated tactile afferents. *Neurosci. Biobehav. Rev.* **2010**, *34*, 185–191. [CrossRef]
160. Monroe, C.M. The effects of therapeutic touch on pain. *J. Holist. Nurs. Off. J. Am. Holist. Nurses' Assoc.* **2009**, *27*, 85–92. [CrossRef]
161. Birznieks, I.; Macefield, V.G.; Westling, G.; Johansson, R.S. Slowly Adapting Mechanoreceptors in the Borders of the Human Fingernail Encode Fingertip Forces. *J. Neurosci.* **2009**, *29*, 9370–9379. [CrossRef]
162. Ebisch, S.J.; Salone, A.; Martinotti, G.; Carlucci, L.; Mantini, D.; Perrucci, M.G.; Saggino, A.; Romani, G.L.; Di Giannantonio, M.; Northoff, G.; et al. Integrative Processing of Touch and Affect in Social Perception: An fMRI Study. *Front. Hum. Neurosci.* **2016**, *10*, 209. [CrossRef]
163. Grion, N.; Akrami, A.; Zuo, Y.; Stella, F.; Diamond, M.E. Coherence between Rat sensorimotor system and hippocampus is enhanced during tactile discrimination. *PLoS Biol.* **2016**, *14*, e1002384. [CrossRef]
164. Macefield, V.G. Physiological characteristics of lowthreshold mechanoreceptors in joints, muscle and skin in human subjects. *Clin. Exp. Pharmacol. Physiol.* **2005**, *32*, 135–144. [CrossRef]
165. Mountcastle, V.C. *The Sensory Hand: Neural Mechanisms of Somatic Sensation*; Harvard University Press: Harvard, MA, USA, 2005.
166. Rushworth, M.F.S.; Paus, T.; Sipila, P.K. Attention systems and the organization of the human parietal cortex. *NeuroImage* **2001**, *13*, 353. [CrossRef]
167. O'Brien, K.M.; Afzal, K.; Tronick, E. Relational psychophysiology and mutual regulation during dyadic therapeutic and developmental relating. In *Interdisciplinary Handbook of the Person-Centered Approach*; Cornelius-White, J., Motschnig-Pitrik, R., Lux, M., Eds.; Springer: New York, NY, USA, 2013; pp. 183–197.

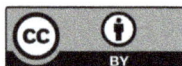

© 2020 by the authors. Licensee MDPI, Basel, Switzerland. This article is an open access article distributed under the terms and conditions of the Creative Commons Attribution (CC BY) license (http://creativecommons.org/licenses/by/4.0/).

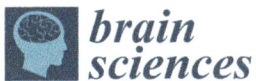

Article

Does the Therapist's Sex Affect the Psychological Effects of Sports Massage?—A Quasi-Experimental Study

Bernhard Reichert [1,2]

1. Institute for Circulatory Research and Sports Medicine, German Sports University Cologne, Am Sportpark Müngersdorf 6, 50933 Köln, Germany; bernhard.reichert@stud.dshs-koeln.de or info@di-uni.de or mail@bernhardreichert.de
2. Public Health and Medicine, Dresden International University, Freiberger. Str. 37, 01067 Dresden, Germany

Received: 18 May 2020; Accepted: 13 June 2020; Published: 16 June 2020

Abstract: Objectives: The aim of this study was to determine the influence of the sex of the therapist and of the athlete on the athlete's current emotional state after a sports massage. The assumption was that the effect of a massage on the current mood was independent of the sex of the therapists or athletes. **Background**: Sports massages are an integral part of the support given to athletes during training or competition and are a commonly used method for promoting athletes' physical and mental recovery. Few studies have measured the mental characteristics or even the nonspecific effects of sports massages. Sexual attraction or dislike are among the nonspecific effects of a treatment. **Materials and methods**: One hundred and sixty-eight high-performance male and female amateur athletes received a sports massage from 15 male and female trained therapists. The current emotional state of the athletes was measured before and after intervention using the BSKE-EA17 adjective scale, whose items can be assigned to five categories of the current emotional state. ANOVAs (analysis of covariances) were carried out to calculate the interactions between the sexes. Cohen's d for similar group sizes and similar group variances were determined. **Results**: Neither the sex of the therapist nor the sex of the athlete had any influence on the mental effect of a sports massage. The only exception was when male athletes were treated by female therapists, where an increase in "elevated mood" was observed. Sports massages resulted in an increase in the responses in the categories "elevated mood" (d = 1.1) and "level of activation" (d = 0.3) and a decrease in the responses for "low mood" (d = 0.3), "level of deactivation" (d = 0.6) and "level of excitation" after the massage compared to before the massage (d = 0.9). **Conclusions**: Sports massages appear to increase the positive dimensions of the athletes' current emotional state and reduce the negative dimensions. The self-reported mood changes from before the massage to after the massage were not influenced by other prognostic variables, including wait time, age of the athlete or the duration of the run. The results suggest that the specific effects of sports massages on the mental status are supported. Disregarding the aspect of the therapists' sex, sports officials, trainers and athletes therefore can be more independent in the personnel planning of sports therapists.

Keywords: sports massage; current emotional state; mood; therapist's sex; athlete's sex

1. Introduction

Massage is the manipulation of soft tissue by a trained therapist as a component of a holistic therapeutic intervention [1,2].

Sports massage is defined as a set of massage techniques that enhance athletes' recovery and help treat pathological conditions [3]. Depending on the time a sports massage is performed in relation to exercise, the terms "pre-event", "pre-exercise", "inter-event", "post-event", "post-exercise" and "training" massage are used [4].

The specific forms of a massage are broken down further into the overall duration, intensity and selection of techniques used. In most studies, technical elements of Swedish, classic or Western massage are used in sports massages: strokes, kneading, petrissage, frictions and vibrations. In the literature, the term "recovery massage" is used to describe a massage delivered after intense exercise [4]. The best outcomes of massages for muscular recovery were achieved when the treatment was applied within the first two hours of exercise [5].

The particular significance of a recovery massage is especially evident in athletes performing repeated exertions within a short period. In athletes competing in multidiscipline events, as well as those participating in various disciplines, top performances must be delivered multiple times on the same day or several days in a row. For this reason, a quick recovery is an important factor for ensuring top performances for the duration of the competition [1].

A sports massage plays a valuable role in the health system [6]. It is an integral component of support for athletes during training or competition. Athletes, those supporting them and individuals associated with sports worldwide recognize sports massages as an effective means of boosting recovery and reducing pain and discomfort [3]. Sports massages are often offered to support athletes at large-scale events. Galloway and Watt reported in 2004 that physical therapists devoted 24.0% to 52.2% of the time they spent supporting athletes at large national and international sports events to massages [7].

Scientific aspects of sports massages are of interest to athletes, their trainers and sports physicians [8]. Schilz and Leach (2020) surveyed 100 endurance athletes about their knowledge regarding the effects of sports massage therapy. Of the athletes surveyed, 93% felt that sports massage therapy could be seen as a form of injury prevention, 92% felt that it was a valuable method of resolving a wide variety of muscular problems and 90% indicated that they felt that sports massage therapy improved their quality of life.

Very few studies have addressed sports massages following endurance performances [9] and very few address psychological factors [9–11]. The latest relevant review by Poppendieck (2016) described the benefits of post-exercise sports massages in detail. These positive effects were observed for strength and endurance exercises, as well as for high-intensity mixed exercises. Since the physiological mechanisms of the performance recovery were unclear for the authors, they described the mental effects as more significant [12].

In general, the study objects, outcomes and results of the different (physiological, in particular) effects of sports massages vary widely, and unequivocal statements are rare [8,13]. Very few studies have measured mental characteristics.

Each therapeutic intervention can be assumed to have an effect component that is directly dependent on the intervention (specific effect) and an effect component that is independent of the intervention (nonspecific effect) [14]. These nonspecific effects include the presence, voice and sex of the therapist; trust; therapeutic alliance [15] and space-related conditions. In order to better classify the value of massage therapy (specific effects), the influences of nonspecific effects on, e.g., mental outcomes should be investigated. No studies are available in the well-known medical databases that investigate the nonspecific effects of a massage with respect to psychological effects [14].

Experience has shown that athletes rarely perceive physical contact occurring during manually applied massages to be unpleasant or anticipate that it will be unpleasant [16]. During the application, one could assume that massage therapy may result in an improved mental status, depending on the sex of the therapist or the athlete, through some kind of sexual stimulation. Culturally formed attitudes may prohibit heterosexual contact between the therapist and the athlete. Negative experiences with heterosexual contact in the personal history of athletes could also lead to preferring a certain sex of the therapist. Therefore, one question that may arise is whether the sex of the therapist or the athlete can contribute to a change in the perception and, thus, contribute to the athlete's assessment of his or her current emotional state. This possible influence has not been investigated in previous studies to date.

The aim of this study was therefore to determine the influence of the sex of the therapist and of the athlete on the athlete's current mental state after a sports massage. The assumption is that the effects of a massage on the current mood is independent of the sex of therapists or athletes. The following research questions led through the study:

(1) In general, does the wellbeing of the athlete change from before the intervention to after the intervention (main effect of time)?
(2) Does the sex of the therapist have a (main) influence on the change in the wellbeing of the athlete?
(3) Does the change of wellbeing depend on the sex of the athlete (so-called interaction effect or interaction)?

2. Materials and Methods

2.1. Participants and Setting

The participants in this quasi-experimental study design were recruited on the day prior to the 19th Stuttgart half-marathon in the city of Stuttgart, Germany. Some 19,000 athletes participated in the race. All of the study participants were ambitious amateur athletes. They were personally approached and encouraged to participate in the study. Recruiting took place in the Hanns-Martin-Schleyer-Halle, a large sports and entertainment venue in Stuttgart. The participants were informed in writing, gave their consent after having read the information and completed a questionnaire to clarify the inclusion/exclusion criteria.

Included in the study were participants in the half-marathon who were between the ages of 18 and 70 and who did not meet any of the exclusion criteria.

Any health condition that negatively impacted the athletes' overall performance capacity—in particular, their running performance, their recovery and the perception of tactile stimuli—were defined as exclusion criteria. They included the following medical criteria:

1. Musculoskeletal system: Disorders of or injuries to muscles, joints or vertebral disks, as well as artificial hip, knee or ankle replacements.
2. Nervous system: Disorders such as polyneuropathy, multiple sclerosis or paralysis.
3. Cardiovascular system: Elevated blood pressure, antihypertensive drugs, heart disease such as arrhythmia, heart failure, heart valve disease, pericarditis or myocarditis.
4. Lungs and respiratory tract: Pulmonary and respiratory disorders and asthma sprays.
5. Renal and metabolism: Renal disorders, kidney transplant and diabetes.

The following variables were recorded as additional prognostic factors:

1. Use of pain-relief medication after the half-marathon.
2. Expected length of the sports massage.
3. Estimated actual length of the sports massage.
4. Influence of the wait time on the current emotional state.
5. Running performance on the race day and weekly training time in the previous three months.

2.1.1. Sample size Calculation

The maximum number of participants was determined based on the number of therapists delivering massages simultaneously (15) and the average duration of the massage therapy. All therapists gave massages continuously and treated as long as there was demand from athletes. All included test persons who visited the massage area were treated.

2.1.2. Assignment of Participants and Blinding

Whenever a massage table freed up, a new athlete was assigned to it, regardless of the sex of either the athlete or the therapist. This means that the male and female athletes were assigned to the male and female therapists in a random fashion, albeit not in the conventional sense. Both male and female athletes participating in the study and male and female athletes not participating in the study underwent massage in the same setting. The participants knew that they were part of a study. The subjects were instructed not to tell the therapists that they were participating in the study, so the therapists were unable to identify these athletes as study participants. The athletes were assigned an ID number, so that the individuals evaluating the questionnaires and those analyzing the data were blinded.

2.2. Study Procedure and Intervention

The participants were requested to come to the massage area on the day of the half-marathon as soon as possible after crossing the finish line. Immediately after they had checked in and before the massage, they filled out a sociodemographic questionnaire and completed a questionnaire about their current emotional state. Immediately after the massage, they completed a second questionnaire about their current emotional state. In terms of the mental outcome variables, there were no differences between the pre-massage and post-massage questionnaires. The participants completed the questionnaires in a separate waiting area within the massage area.

The massages were delivered near the finish area of the half-marathon in a separate area in which 15 massage tables were set up next to each other without any partitions. Participants and athletes not participating in the study were treated identically and were assigned to a free massage table.

The massage therapists (8 male and 7 female) were students enrolled in the physical therapy school in Fellbach, Germany and were trained for several hours to perform the sports massage standardized in duration, techniques, sequence and intensity. The massage length was set at 15 to 20 min. The massage entailed the treatment of two legs only with the techniques used in classic massage therapy: strokes, kneading, petrissage and frictions, with the balls of the hands on the front and back of the legs. This corresponds to the way a sports massage is performed on endurance athletes [16] and the way sports massages were conducted in previous studies by the author [17]. A neutral commercially available massage oil without any additives was used for the massage. All of the sports massages took place on the same day between approximately 11:00 a.m. and 4:00 p.m.

2.3. Measurement Instruments

In addition to a sociodemographic questionnaire with additional prognostic variables, a questionnaire for describing the athlete's current mental state was used. The latter questionnaire comprised a short form of the adjective list compiled by Janke, Erdmann and Hüppe (BSKE-EA 17), which was used in various previous studies [18]. This 17-item scale was suitable for recording the respondents' current emotional states and any short-term changes. The items were assigned to different categories:

1. Elevated mood, three items: emotional wellbeing, feeling of being relaxed and feeling of joy
2. Low mood, five items: dysphoric feeling, feeling anxious, feeling sad, feeling angry and feeling physically unwell
3. Level of activation, two items: feeling of being active and feeling of alertness
4. Deactivation, two items: lack of energy and feeling tired
5. Level of excitement, four items: feeling of inner excitement, feeling of physical excitement, feeling of shakiness and feeling of inner tension

Mood in psychology is a form of pleasant or unpleasant feeling that forms the background of human experiences. Mood depends on the (biological) overall constitution of the individual and the individual's current emotional state [19].

Janke and Debus described some of these categories in their manual [20] as follows:

Activation: "State-of-mind feature characterized by pleasure-oriented activity that is primarily performance-oriented but also environmentally oriented [...] and encompasses holistically somatic and psychological aspects of activity." A high rating for activation describes a state of the highest possible performance efficiency and wellbeing.

Deactivation: "State-of-mind feature characterized by reduced activity with respect to performance and the environment (relation to introversion!). This reduced activity is closely connected to the feeling of overall impaired willingness and ability to perform in the sense that the individual feels a lack of ability and lack of willingness to do anything."

Excitement: "State-of-mind feature characterized by motor restlessness and tension characterized by lack of desire and emotional disequilibrium (emotional lability), combined with performance inefficiency."

Each description of the current emotional state (item) could be evaluated using a Likert scale in seven gradations. These items were coded between 0 = "not at all" and 6 = "very strong". The participants used this instrument to evaluate themselves and indicate to what extent certain feeling states corresponded to their current emotional states. Each scale is marked by a noun and two exemplary adjectives (see example in Figure 1).

10. Feeling of **alertness** (e.g., attentive, alert)						
0	1	2	3	4	5	6
Not at all	Very weak	Weak	Somewhat strong	Rather strong	Strong	Very strong

Figure 1. Example of an item from the BSKE-EA 17 scale with gradation and coding.

This yields the following point ranges for each category: elevated mood (0 to 18 points), low mood (0 to 30 points), activation (0 to 12 points), deactivation (0 to 12 points) and excitement (0 to 24 points). Totaling the scores of these scales would not be expedient, which is why the items were evaluated by category.

2.4. Objectives and Outcomes

The primary outcome of this study was to describe the influence of the therapist's sex and of the participant's sex on the psychological effects of a sports massage. It was assumed that neither the sex of the therapist nor that of the athlete would have an effect.

The secondary research question was as follows: What general effect does a sports massage have on an athlete's current state of mind? Do any other prognostic factors (wait time until the massage, age of the athlete or duration of the race) have an influence?

A positive influence on the part of the sports massage on the athlete's current state of mind is considered to be an increase in the responses in the categories "elevated mood" and "activation" and a decrease in the responses for "low mood", "deactivation" and "excitement".

2.5. Statistical Methods

The data were recorded in MS Excel [21] and prepared for analysis in IBM SPSS 19.0 [22]. A questionnaire was excluded if more than one item of the outcome variables was not filled out. All other missing values were replaced by mean values. Calculating a total score for the multidimensional emotional state questionnaire (BSKE_EA 17) would not be expedient, which is why the items were evaluated by category. The Kolmogorov-Smirnov test was used to test the metric variables for normal distribution.

T-tests for dependent samples were calculated to statistically test the before-and-after differences. The differences in effects between men and women were calculated using the t-test for independent samples. To analyze the effects of the sex of the therapist and the effects of the sex of the athlete on the change in the five scales of T1 (pre-massage) to T2 (post-massage), the effect size for mean differences (Cohens d) between two groups (before and after the sports massage) was calculated with similar group sizes and similar group variances. The interpretation of the effect size was based on [23]: low effect size = 0.1 to 0.2, medium effect size = 0.3 to 0.5 and large effect size >0.5.

Mixed ANOVAs were conducted to evaluate the effects of the therapist's sex and the athlete's sex on the changes in the five dependent categories (scales). Furthermore, ANOVAs (analysis of covariances) were carried out. In this context, the following hypotheses were tested:

(1) The sex of the therapist has a (main) effect on the change in wellbeing.
(2) This effect is dependent on the sex of the athlete ("interaction effect").
(3) In general, wellbeing will change from T1 to T2 (main effect of time).

To study the influence of the interval-scaled variables "wait time", "running performance" (in minutes) and "age" on the change from T1 to T2, multiple regression analyses were performed with the difference values of T2 and T1 as dependent variables. This thus allowed us to investigate whether, for example, shorter wait times were associated with higher difference values (= stronger changes from before to after the massages).

3. Results

3.1. Deviations from the Protocol

No motivated participants were excluded for health-related reasons before inclusion in the study. No participants discontinued their participation in the study, and no adverse effects of the massages were observed.

3.2. Participants' Characteristics

In all, 200 athletes were recruited—of whom, 185 athletes were included in the study and underwent a sports massage as planned. Seventeen questionnaires were excluded from evaluation owing to missing responses. The responses of 127 male athletes and 41 female athletes were evaluated. Table 1 shows the athletes' characteristics. They were, on average, 37 years old, approx. 178 cm tall and had a BMI of approx. 23. They had trained for an average of 32 km a week in the previous three months and achieved an average race time of 1:50:55 (h:mm:ss) for the half-marathon distance on the race day. The participants estimated the optimum time taken for a sports massage after a half-marathon at an average of 21 min and estimated the perceived duration of the massage they underwent at 12 min. They waited six minutes on average from the time they entered the massage area to the onset of the sports massage (see Table 1). Seventy-two point two percent reported that the wait time prior to the onset of the sports massage did not negatively influence their current emotional state. Nine athletes (5.7%) took medication prior to the competition that could have an influence on their recovery and current state (e.g., aspirin or diclofenac). The participants received 80 massages by male therapists and 88 massages by female therapists.

Table 1. Participant characteristics. MV = mean value, Med = median, SD = standard deviation, Min = minimum, Max = maximum and BMI = body mass index.

Characteristic	MV	Med	SD	Min	Max
Age (in years)/all	37.10	37.00	±10.16	18	69
male	37.75	37.00	±10.27	18	69
female	35.10	35.00	±9.56	18	59
BMI/all	23.11	22.99	±2.51	18.00	30.87
male	23.72	23.55	±2.35	17.65	30.87
female	21.19	21.05	±1.99	15.22	25.71
Running time (h:mm:ss)/all	01:50:55	01:49:00	00:18:20	01:01:00	02:57:00
male	01:47:57	01:48:00	00:17:07	01:19:00	02:57:00
female	02:00:50	02:03:00	00:18:45	01:01:00	02:36:00
Training (km)/all	31.91	25.00	±37.25	0	350
male	34.67	30.00	±41.81	0	350
female	23.35	25.00	±13.16	3	50
Estimated Massage duration (received, in min)/all	11.94	10.00	±4.10	1	20
male	12.01	10.00	±4.22	1	20
female	11.73	10.00	±3.69	5	20
Estimated Wait time (in min)	5.86	5.00	±9.55	0	78
male	6.55	5.00	±1.,76	0	78
female	3.73	3.00	±3.04	0	15.00

3.3. Results of the Outcome Variables

Table 2 shows the descriptive analysis for the outcome variables or the before-after comparisons differentiated by group. Sports massages resulted in an increase in the responses in the categories "elevated mood" (d = 1.1) and "activation" (d = 0.3) and a decrease in the responses for "low mood" (d = 0.4), "deactivation" (d = 0.6) and "excitation" after the massage compared to before the massage (d = 0.9). Testing the differences in the results of women and men before and after applications with the two-tailed t-test for independent samples revealed a p-value <0.05 only for the category "excitement" after the treatment. Table 3 presents the results of the analytical statistics for the outcome variables for the before-after comparisons, differentiated by group.

Table 2. Descriptive data for the outcome variables. Mean value (standard deviation) and Diff = difference.

Category	Before/All	Bevor/Male	Bevor/Female	After/All	After/Male	After/Female	Diff/All	Diff/Male	Diff/Female
Elevated mood	10.88 (±2.49)	10.99 (±2.48)	10.51 (±2.50)	13.63 (±2.45)	13.71 (±2.47)	13.39 (±2.37)	2.76 (±2.58)	2.72 (±2.70)	2.88 (±2.17)
Low mood	3.44 (±3.94)	3.71 (±4.27)	2.61 (±2.46)	2.14 (±3.61)	2.31 (±3.85)	1.61 (±2.67)	1.30 (±3.00)	1.39 (±3.16)	1.00 (±2.41)
Activation	6.14 (±1.94)	6.27 (±1.87)	5.73 (±2,07)	6.81 (±1.94)	6.96 (±1.87)	6.34 (±2.08)	0.67 (±2.13)	0.69 (±2.11)	0.61 (±2.20)
Deactivation	5.55 (±2.42)	5.62 (±2.51)	5.32 (±2,13)	4.26 (±2.38)	4.17 (±2.46)	4.51 (±2.10)	1.29 (±2.17)	1.45 (±2.01)	0.80 (±2.54)
Excitement	5.98 (±3.61)	6.02 (±3.72)	5.49 (±3,25)	3.43 (±3.24)	3.80 (±3.38)	2.27 (±2.42)	2.46 (±2.80)	2.21 (±2.75)	3.22 (±2.80)

Table 3. Analytical statistics for the outcome variables; d = Cohen's d and p = P-value.

Cohen's d and p-Values for the Differences the Outcome Variables						
	d/All	d/Male	d/Female	p-Value/All	p-Value/Male	p-Value/Female
Elevated mood	1.1	1.0	1.3	<0.001	<0.001	<0.001
Low mood	0.3	0.4	0.4	<0.001	<0.001	<0.001
Activation	0.3	0.3	0.3	<0.001	<0.001	=0.0434
Deactivation	0.6	0.7	0.3	<0.001	<0.001	=0.0259
Excitement	0.9	0.8	1.2	<0.001	<0.001	<0.001

ANOVAs were conducted to evaluate the effects of the therapist's sex and the athlete's sex on the changes in the five dependent categories (scales) between T1 and T2 (Table 4). The resulting design was a 2 (therapist's sex: male vs. female) × 2 (athlete's sex: male vs. female) × 2 (time: T1 vs. T2) mixed factorial, with time as a repeated measures factor.

Table 4. Results of the mixed ANOVA.

	Elevated Mood	Low Mood	Activation	Deactivation	Excitement
time	$F(1.164) = 146.4$ $p < 0.001$ $\eta_p^2 = 0.47$	$F(1.164) = 18.8$ $p < 0.001$ $\eta_p^2 = 0.10$	$F(1.163) = 11.8$ $p = 0.001$ $\eta_p^2 = 0.07$	$F(1.163) = 33.1$ $p = 0.001$ $\eta_p^2 = 0.17$	$F(1.165) = 116.9$ $p = 0.001$ $\eta_p^2 = 0.42$
sex T	$F(1.164) = 0.07$ $p = 0.79$ $\eta_p^2 < 0.01$	$F(1.164) = 1.2$ $p = 0.28$ $\eta_p^2 < 0.01$	$F(1.163) = 0.3$ $p = 0.57$ $\eta_p^2 < 0.01$	$F(1.163) = 2.3$ $p = 0.13$ $\eta_p^2 = 0.01$	$F(1.165) = 3.3$ $p = 0.07$ $\eta_p^2 < 0.02$
sex A	$F(1.164) = 0.92$ $p = 0.34$ $\eta_p^2 < 0.01$	$F(1.164) = 2.6$ $p = 0.14$ $\eta_p^2 = 0.01$	$F(1,163) = 4.4$ $p = 0.04$ $\eta_p^2 = 0.03$	$F(1.163) = 0.0$ $p = 0.98$ $\eta_p^2 < 0.01$	$F(1.165) = 4.0$ $p < 0.05$ $\eta_p^2 = 0.02$
time x sex T	$F(1.164) = 2.1$ $p = 0.15$ $\eta_p^2 = 0.01$	$F(1.164) = 0.6$ $p = 0.43$ $\eta_p^2 = <0.01$	$F(1.163) = 0.0$ $p = 0.90$ $\eta_p^2 < 0.01$	$F(1.163) = 3.1$ $p = 0.08$ $\eta_p^2 < 0.02$	$F(1.165) = 0.4$ $p = 0.56$ $\eta_p^2 < 0.01$
sex T x sex A	$F(1.164) = 4.21$ $p = 0.04$ $\eta_p^2 < 0.01$	$F(1.164) = 0.5$ $p = 0.47$ $\eta_p^2 < 0.01$	$F(1.163) = 0.1$ $p = 0.73$ $\eta_p^2 < 0.01$	$F(1.163) = 1.0$ $p = 0.32$ $\eta_p^2 < 0.01$	$F(1.165) = 1.7$ $p = 0.20$ $\eta_p^2 < 0.01$
time x sex T x sex A	$F(1.164) < 0.01$ $p = 0.96$ $\eta_p^2 < 0.01$	$F(1.164) = 1.0$ $p = 0.31$ $\eta_p^2 < 0.01$	$F(1.163) < 0.0$ $p = 0.99$ $\eta_p^2 < 0.01$	$F(1.163) = 5.0$ $p = 0.03$ $\eta_p^2 = 0.03$	$F(1.165) = 0.7$ $p = 0.39$ $\eta_p^2 < 0.01$

Time: main effect of time, sex A: effect of sex of the athlete, sex T: effect of sex of the therapist, time x sex T: two-way interaction of time and sex of the therapist, sex A x sex T: two-way interaction of sex of the therapist and sex of the athlete and time x sex A x sex T: three-way interaction of time, sex of the therapist and sex of the athlete. F: test of equality of variances, η_p^2: Partial Eta Squared.

Some comments on some dependent categories:

- Activation
  Of all the other effects, only the main effect of sex of the athlete was significant, $F(1.163) = 4.4$, $p = 0.04$ and $\eta_p^2 = 0.03$, indicating that males reported overall higher levels of "activation" than females.
- Deactivation
  Paired post-hoc (LSD) comparisons showed that the decrease in "deactivation" was significant for almost all combinations of the sex of the athletes and sex of the therapists, all $p < 0.01$, but not for female athletes who received a massage from a male therapist ($p = 0.59$).
- Excitement
  Paired post-hoc (LSD) comparisons showed that the male and female athletes did not differ in their levels of "excitement" before the massage, $p = 0.36$, but after the massage, male athletes reported significantly higher levels of "excitement" than female athletes, $p < 0.01$, albeit lower than before the massage.
- Effects of wait time, athlete's age and duration of the run
  To analyze the effects of wait time, age of the athlete and duration of the run (time in minutes), regression analyses were conducted with these variables, as prognostic variables and difference scores of the questionnaire scales before and after the massage were used as dependent variables. None of the five regression analyses yielded a significant effect of any of the three prognostic variables.

The hypotheses set out above can be answered as follows:

Hypothesis 1: *In general, the current mood changed from T1 to T2 (main effect of time). This hypothesis can be accepted. The low mood decreased significantly from the time before to the time after the massage, regardless of the sex of the therapist or athlete. The feeling of activation increased significantly from the time before to the time after the massage and was greater in men than in women, regardless of the sex of the therapist or athlete.*

In summary, almost all athletes showed a significant decrease in the feeling of deactivation from the time before to the time after the massage, with the exception of the group of female athletes who were massaged by male therapists. In this group, the feeling of deactivation after the massage was no different. The level of arousal decreased significantly as a result of the sports massage, although male athletes reported significantly higher "arousal levels" than female athletes, although lower than before the massage.

Hypothesis 2: *The sex of the therapist had a (main) effect on changes in the current mood. This hypothesis must generally be rejected.*

Hypothesis 3: *The change in the current mood depended on the sex of the athlete ("interaction effect"). This hypothesis must generally be rejected. The only relevant difference found in the study regarding the influence of the sex of the therapist or the athlete was that both before and after the massage, male athletes reported significantly better moods than female athletes when the male athletes received a massage from a female therapist. All other interactions between the sex of the therapist and the sex of the athlete were not significant.*

4. Discussion

A total of 185 recruited athletes in the study—of whom, the data of 168 ambitious amateur athletes were evaluated. Fifteen trained students performed the post-exercise massages after a half-marathon. The participant characteristics data corresponded to a survey conducted in 2011 that recorded the data at the same location as the same event and with the same intervention [17].

The aim of this research was to show whether the sex of the therapist or the athlete had an influence on the mental effects of a sports massage and whether the mental state improved with the treatment. In summary, the athletes reported a significantly higher positive and decreased negative mental state after the massage than prior to the massage, and this effect was, in general, identical regardless of the sex of either the therapist or the athlete. The only exception was when male athletes were treated by female therapists, where an increase in "elevated mood" was observed. These results are nearly all congruent with the results of studies addressing the mental recovery of athletes undergoing post-exercise sports massages [9–11,16,17]. Hemmings et al. (2000) employed a pre-/post-design to study the physiological and psychological effects of recovery massages in boxers. They showed that the boxers reported a significantly increased perception of recovery after a massage than after passive resting [11]. In a randomized, controlled design involving 108 half-marathon participants, Reichert, 2011 showed that a sports massage significantly increased the elevated mood and reduced the low mood compared to passive resting [17].

In general, too few studies have been conducted with mental outcomes to attest to a fundamental unequivocal effect of sports massages, regardless of athletic discipline. The present study showed that the influence of sex plays, at most, a negligible role with regards to short-term mental outcomes.

5. Conclusions

To our knowledge, this was the first study of the nonspecific effects of the sex of therapists and athletes during a massage treatment on their mental status. The study showed that neither the therapist's sex nor the athlete's sex influenced the mental effects of the sports massage. Sports massages appear to increase the positive dimensions of the athletes' current emotional states and reduce the negative dimensions. The self-reported mood changes from before the massages to after the massages were not influenced by other prognostic variables, including the wait time, age of the athlete or the duration of the run. The results suggest supporting the specific effects of sports massages on the mental status. The question of sex is clearly irrelevant to the outcome. Sports officials, trainers and athletes can therefore be more independent in the personnel planning of sports therapists.

In the future, additional studies with a similar study design should be carried out that include control groups and focus on other sports disciplines, as well as on professional athletes. The influence of the therapist's/athlete's sex on the mental outcomes should also be investigated for other types of massage (e.g., classic massage) and treatment settings (e.g., rehabilitation). Furthermore, the other nonspecific effects of treatments on these outcomes must also be examined.

6. Limitations

Cohen's d was calculated in the study because no comparable data for classifying the effect size was available from previous studies. For the differences between T1 (pre-massage) and T2 (post-sports massage), however, it should be noted that the lack of a control group meant that, principally, no causal interpretation was possible that would allow the difference to be attributed to the massage. However, in a similar study with a randomized controlled design by Reichert (2011), a significant advantage of sports massage vs. passive rest with regards to the current mental state was suggested [17].

Author Contributions: Conceptualization, methodology, formal analysis, resources, writing, supervision by the autor. The author have read and agreed to the published version of the manuscript.

Funding: This research received no external funding.

Acknowledgments: I would like to thank the students at the VPT Akademie staatl, anerk, Massageschule Fellbach for their hands-on support and the Württembergische Leichtathletik Verband (track and field association) for logistical support with implementing this study.

Conflicts of Interest: There are no conflicts of interest. The entire study protocol and all data may be obtained from the author.

References

1. Holey, E.C.E. *Evidence-Based Therapeutic Massage. A Practical Guide for Therapists*, 3rd ed.; Elsevier Ltd.: Edinburgh, UK, 2011.
2. Weerapong, P.; Hume, P.A.; Kolt, G.S. The mechanisms of massage and effects on performance, muscle recovery and injury prevention. *Sport. Med.* **2005**, *35*, 235–256. [CrossRef] [PubMed]
3. Sinha, A. *Principles and Practice of Therapeutic Massage*, 2nd ed.; Jaypee Brothers Medical Publishers LTD.: St Louis, MO, USA, 2010.
4. Angus, S. Massage therapy for sprinters and runners. *Clin. Podiatr. Med. Surg.* **2001**, *18*, 329–336. [PubMed]
5. Best, T.M.; Hunter, R.; Wilcox, A.; Haq, F. Effectiveness of sports massage for recovery of skeletal muscle from strenuous exercise. *Clin. J. Sport Med.* **2008**, *18*, 446–460. [CrossRef] [PubMed]
6. Shroff, F.M.; Sahota, I.S. The perspectives of educators, regulators and funders of massage therapy on the state of the profession in British Columbia, Canada. *Chiropr. Man. Therap.* **2013**, *21*, 2. [CrossRef] [PubMed]
7. Galloway, S.D.R.; Watt, J.M. Massage provision by physiotherapists at major athletics events between 1987 and 1998. *Br. J. Sports Med.* **2004**, *38*, 235–236. [CrossRef] [PubMed]
8. Moraska, A. Sports massage: A comprehensive review. *J. Sports Med. Phys. Fit.* **2005**, *45*, 370–380.
9. Hemmings, B.J. Physiological, psychological and performance effects of massage therapy in sport: A review of the literature. *Phys. Ther. Sport* **2001**, *2*, 165–170. [CrossRef]
10. Dawson, L.G.; Dawson, K.A.; Tiidus, P.M. Evaluating the influence of massage on leg strength, swelling, and pain following a half-marathon. *J. Sport. Sci. Med.* **2004**, *3*, 37–43.
11. Hemmings, B.; Smith, M.; Graydon, J.; Dyson, R. Effects of massage on physiological restoration, perceived recovery, and repeated sports performance. *Br. J. Sports Med.* **2000**, *34*, 109–114. [CrossRef] [PubMed]
12. Poppendieck, W.; Wegmann, M.; Ferrauti, A.; Kellmann, M.; Pfeiffer, M.; Meyer, T. Massage and Performance Recovery: A Meta-Analytical Review. *Sports Med.* **2016**, *46*, 183–204. [CrossRef] [PubMed]
13. Hart, J.M.; Swanik, C.B.; Tierney, R.T. Effects of sport massage on limb girth and discomfort associated with eccentric exercise. *J. Athl. Train.* **2005**, *40*, 181–185. [PubMed]
14. Reichert, B. *Massage-Therapie*; Thieme: Stuttgart, Germany, 2015.
15. Horvath, A.O.; Luborsky, L. The role of the therapeutic alliance in psychotherapy. *J. Consult. Clin. Psychol.* **1993**, *61*, 561–573. [CrossRef] [PubMed]
16. Schilz, M.; Leach, L. Knowledge and Perception of Athletes on Sport Massage Therapy (SMT). *Int. J. Ther. Massage Bodyw.* **2020**, *13*, 13–21.
17. Reichert, B. *Psychological Effects of a Regeneration Massage for Half Marathon Runners*; University of Applied Sciences Vienna: Wien, Austria, 2011.

18. Janke, W.; Erdmann, G.; Hüppe, M.; Debus, G. *Befindlichkeitsskalierung Anhand von Kategorien und Eigenschaftswörterlisten BSKE*; Julius-Maximilians-Universität Würzburg: Würzburg, Germany, 1999.
19. Arnold, W.; Eysenck, H.; Meili, R. *Lexikon der Psychologie*, 3rd ed.; Herder Verlag: Freiburg/Basel/Wien, Germany, 1972.
20. Janke, W.; Debus, G. *Die Eigenschaftswörterliste EWL*; Handanweisung, Hogrefe Verlag für Psychologie: Göttingen, Germany, 1978.
21. Microsoft Corporation, Redmond, WA 98052-6399, U. Microsoft Corporation, Redmond, WA 98052-6399, USA.
22. *IBM Deutschland GmbH, Statistical Package for the Social Sciences (SPSS®)*; Version 19; IBM: Ehningen, Germany, 2018.
23. Cohen, J. *Statistical Power Analysis for the Behavioral Sciences*, 2nd ed.; L. Erlbaum Associates: Hillsdale, NJ, USA, 1988; ISBN 0-8058-0283-5.

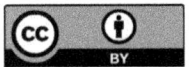

© 2020 by the author. Licensee MDPI, Basel, Switzerland. This article is an open access article distributed under the terms and conditions of the Creative Commons Attribution (CC BY) license (http://creativecommons.org/licenses/by/4.0/).

MDPI
St. Alban-Anlage 66
4052 Basel
Switzerland
Tel. +41 61 683 77 34
Fax +41 61 302 89 18
www.mdpi.com

Brain Sciences Editorial Office
E-mail: brainsci@mdpi.com
www.mdpi.com/journal/brainsci

www.ingramcontent.com/pod-product-compliance
Lightning Source LLC
LaVergne TN
LVHW070542100526
838202LV00012B/352